I dedicate this book to those who choose not to confuse activity with accomplishment.

TRISOmetrics™

Advanced Strength Training and Muscle Building

Published by

MajorVision International

2018

Approved by The World Isometric Exercise Association
www.TWiEA.com

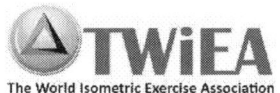

Copyright and Trademark Notice
© 2018 Brian Sterling-Vete and Helen Renée Wuorio All Rights Reserved

All material in this book is the property of, copyright, and trademarked to Brian Sterling-Vete and Helen Renée Wuorio, and/or MajorVision Ltd, unless otherwise stated; AE&OE. Copyright and other intellectual property laws protect these materials. Reproduction, distribution, or transmission of the materials, in whole or in part, in any manner, without the prior written consent of the copyright holder is prohibited and is a violation of national and international copyright law.

The following names, exercises, and workout systems are the property of, copyright, and trademarked to Brian Sterling-Vete and Helen Renée, and/or MajorVision Ltd. ISOfitness™, The 70 Second Difference™, Adaptive Response™, The 1664 Workout™, The 1664 Workout Challenge™, Zero Footprint Workout™, ZFW™, Fitness on the Move™, FOM™, The ISO90™ Course, ISO90™, The SSASS Workout™, SSASS™, Dynamic Flexation™, The Bullworker Bible™, The Bullworker 90™, The Bullworker Compendium™, Workout at Work™, Doorway to Strength™, TRISOmetric™, TRISOmetrics™, The ISOmetric Bible™, Brian Sterling-Vete's Mental Martial Arts™, Tuxedo Warriors™, The Tuxedo Warrior™, The Pike™, The Beast of Kane™, Being American Married to a Brit, and Paranormal Investigation - The Black Book of Scientific Ghost Hunting and How to Investigate Paranormal Phenomena™, The Haunting of Lilford Hall™.

Artwork and design: **WWW.MAJORVISION.COM**
www.MajorVision.com

Contents

Important General Safety and Health Guidelines

1. **Different Types of Exercise**
    - Different Types of Muscle Contraction
    - Callisthenics
    - Isokinetic Training
    - Isometrics
    - The Science
2. **Strength at Only One Angle?**
    - Supination and Strong Arms
    - Super-Slow Training
3. **The TRISOmetric™ Exercise Concept**
4. **Workout Intensity**
    - Ultra-High Intensity, Ultra-Short Burst™
    - Strength, Stamina, Endurance, and Resilience
    - Rest and Recovery
    - Dynamic Flexation™
    - What is ISOfitness™ and TWiEA™?
    - The 70 Second Difference™ Book
    - TWiEA™ Resources
5. **The Iso-Bow® and Other Devices**
    - The Iso-Bow®
    - Securing the Iso-Bow® With Your Feet
    - The Bow Extension®
    - Extending the Iso-Bow® and Bow Extension®
    - The Iso-Gym®
    - The Bullworker®
    - The Steel Bow®
    - Other Equipment and Techniques
6. **Things to Remember Before You Begin**
    - Important Notes About Exercise Equipment and Choices
7. **TRISOmetric Exercises**
    - Things to Remember
    - Warm up and Cool Down
8. **Conclusion**

Important General Safety and Health Guidelines

This section entitled, "Important General Safety and Health Guidelines," pertains to The ISOfitness™ Exercise System, and all books and publications about it not limited to but including The ISO90™ Course, Fitness on the Move™, The 70 Second Difference™, The Bullworker Bible™, the Sixty Second Ass Workout™, The Bullworker 90™ Course, The Bullworker Compendium™, Workout at Work™, The Doorway to Strength™, TRISOmetrics™, TRISOmetric™, the TRISOmetric™ system, ISOmetrics, The ISOmetric Bible™, the Iso-Bow® System, recommendations, suggestions, coaching, and advice, either written, verbal, in audio format, on video, written, or given, implied, or suggested the authors, from Brian Sterling-Vete, Helen Renée Wuorio, and the works thereof.

You should never begin any kind of sport, exercise system, workout plan, or diet modification, including everything contained in this book and in any books mentioned in the beginning paragraph above unless you have consulted with and have the full approval of your medical doctor.

Your physician can properly assess your current health status, and your ability to perform the exercises in the book and/or course. This is particularly important if you have any known or unknown pre-existing health issues, if you're pregnant, or if you believe that you may have other serious health conditions.

It's essential that you must always have the absolute approval from your physician before starting. Please show all the material in the above courses, books, video/audio, online material, and their content to your physician and get their approval before you start.

All exercises, suggestions, recommendations, instructions, exercise plans, dietary and eating recommendations, either given or implied, are intended only as a reference, and they are no substitute for a qualified professional personal coach who can help you to plan an exercise and diet program appropriate for your age and physical condition. Never overexert yourself when performing any exercise.

Stop exercising immediately and consult your doctor if you ever experience any pain, irregular heartbeat, shortness of breath, tightness in your chest/arms/fingers, faintness, nausea, or feelings of dizziness. Then consult your doctor and/or call the EMS immediately.

The exercises, courses, plans, and dietary recommendations in this book together with all those mentioned in all the books, general publications, online material, and videos mentioned in the names in paragraph 1 of this section, are not intended for use by children. Keep all exercise equipment out of the reach of children.

Always inspect any exercise equipment, and/or any/all other improvised or specifically made exercise equipment/materials, doors, door jambs, and door frames, and anything else you use before each use to ensure its proper operation and to ensure that it is undamaged and safe. Do not use it unless all parts are free from wear, and it is functioning properly. To avoid serious injury, care should always be taken using any/all exercise equipment, and in all items, people, books and courses, mentioned in paragraph 1 of this section.

Care should always be taken when getting into all exercise positions, on and off the floor, on and off chairs, on and off benches, on and off any other surface that might be used for exercise, including pieces of furniture, and in the use of all exercised equipment, either purpose made or improvised.

The creators, writers, instructors, originators, and owners of The Bullworker90™ Course, The ISO90 Course™, TRISOmetrics™, and all other courses, publications on video, audio, and in print, together with the courses, and websites, owned, originated, and created by the copyright holders and the ISOfitness™ team, including all books, courses, and people mentioned in paragraph 1 of this section, accept no responsibility whatsoever for any injury, harm, damage, illness, harm, damage to property, or any other negative health-related condition which may occur as a direct, or indirect result of following these courses, recommendations, suggestions, diagrams, pictures, videos, or while performing any exercises in these or any related other related material/publication/s.

For additional general information, we also recommend that you check reputable accredited medical advice sites, such as the two listed below.

The National Health Service in the United Kingdom, online at: https://www.nhs.uk/Livewell/fitness/pages/physical-activity-guidelines-for-adults.aspx

In the USA, The Mayo Clinic online: http://www.mayoclinic.org/healthy-lifestyle/fitness/in-depth/exercise/art-20047414

Chapter 1: Different Types of Exercise

All muscle training falls into three categories. These are isotonic training, isokinetic training and isometric training. Isotonic training is all about movement with muscle shortening and lengthening during the lifting and lowering phases of exercise. Isokinetic training is about movement too, however, no matter how much force is applied during an isokinetic exercise, the speed of movement always remains constant. Finally, there is isometric training where there is no movement at all during an exercise. During an isometric exercise, a muscle is pitted against an immovable object under constant force for a between 7 and 10 seconds.

Different Types of Muscle Contraction

There are three different types of muscle contraction. These are a concentric contraction which is the lifting phase of an exercise when the muscles shorten in length, the eccentric phase which is the lowering part of an exercise when the muscles lengthen, and an isometric contraction where the muscle neither lengthens or shortens because it remains at a fixed point during the entire phase of the exercise.

Callisthenics

Just like weight training, callisthenics are a form of isotonic training. There are several methods of exercise that are a viable satisfactory alternative to a traditional gym-based exercise routine. The first that comes to mind is a basic freehand callisthenic routine. A callisthenic routine simply means bodyweight-only exercises of various kinds, such as push-ups, pull-ups, squats, lunges, trunk curls, and dips etc. The word "callisthenics" is derived from a combination of the ancient Greek words "kalos," which means "perfect," and "sthenos," meaning "strength."

These exercises are excellent at building and maintaining high levels of fitness, balance, endurance, and a considerable degree of strength. There are certain callisthenic exercises which can develop great strength, such as the ones used by gymnasts. These are primarily pull-ups, dips, and handstand dips.

During the gymnastic-style exercises, the gymnast performing them would adjust the speed, velocity, and the angles that the exercise is typically performed at, which usually significantly increases their difficulty. These exercises almost always include a portion of isometric, or static, exercise-holds as well.

There is a serious drawback to advanced callisthenics being a complete substitute for a gym-based strength workout. This is that for most people without excellent gymnastic skills, once you've become accustomed to handling your own bodyweight when performing the various exercises, then you need to use techniques to place you at a biomechanical disadvantage to gain increased resistance.

In addition, you need a certain degree of equipment available, and/or similarly improvised facilities to allow a gymnastic-style workout routine to be performed. At the very least, you'll need equipment or facilities to perform pull-ups and dips. If you don't have these, then unless you find another way of applying more resistance through biomechanical disadvantage during each exercise, then you're primarily only performing a basic fitness/resilience/endurance routine. You're almost certainly not performing a resistance routine that is focussed on growing strength and muscle. The other major drawback is that you need a certain degree of space to perform an effective gymnastic-style callisthenics workout routine. Therefore, you can't really perform any exercise easily, and relatively unobtrusively in a public or semi-public place.

Instead of callisthenics, is there another alternative and effective way to exercise? An exercise method that delivers similar, or often even greater benefits than traditional weight training as a gym does? An exercise system that takes much less time to perform and that can be performed almost anywhere? An exercise method that only requires the bare minimum of equipment and that uses quite possibly the world's most compact total-body gym that can easily fit into your pocket?

Isokinetic Training

Isokinetic is a type of calisthenic exercise, or exercise involving movement, that takes place at a constant speed no matter how much effort is exerted. The word, "isokinetic" comes from a combination of ancient Greek and Latin. The word "Isos" means: same/equal, and the word "kinesis" means motion or movement.

One of the main advantages of isokinetic exercise is that the muscles being exercised gain strength evenly throughout the full range of movement of the limb being exercised. Also, a great deal of research suggests that isokinetic training is one of the most efficient ways to increase strength and build muscle. This could also be due, at least in part, to the slower exercise speeds being used while generating maximum tension/force for each repetition of an exercise.

One of the typical disadvantages of isokinetic training is that it typically requires special exercise equipment that is very expensive. This is because the equipment has to sense when a movement is increasing in speed so that it then automatically increases the resistance in order to slow it down and maintain the desired constant speed for the exercise. To a certain degree, the development and implementation of the off-set elliptical cams in most modern exercise machines are a less expensive, but much less efficient way of addressing this issue.

Isometrics

Isometric exercise does not involve any movement. Instead, the joint angle and the muscle length do not change during contraction. An isometric exercise pits a muscle against an immovable object to engage as many muscle fibres as possible in a maximum muscular contraction. Each exercise takes between only 7 and 10 seconds to perform, and ideally, it only requires two small pieces of equipment. The exercise equipment needed is called an Iso-Bow®. Even a pair of them are so compact that they can easily fit into the average jacket pocket, or jeans pocket, they can easily fit into a handbag, an average purse, or a briefcase.

More importantly, with a pair of Iso-Bows®, you can effectively exercise every major muscle group of the body. The level of workout you can get from using a pair of Iso-Bows® can range from an easy, low-level beginner's workout, right up to a very high-intensity professional athlete level of workout. Amazingly, you can do all of this without any adjustment being needed to the Iso-Bows®. Each user will benefit proportionately, according to the amount of effort and intensity that is applied during each exercise.

A simple 7-exercise workout routine, such as one from "The 70 Second Difference" book, will exercise every major muscle of the body in a single session. More importantly, it will only take between 49 and 70 seconds of consecutive exercise time to perform if you take no break whatsoever between exercises. This isn't typically possible for most people, however, even factoring-in a full 1-minute break-time between each exercise, adding a total of 7 minutes of rest-time to the overall workout, it still means that your total-body exercise session will be completed in between only 7 minutes and 49 seconds/469 seconds, or 8 minutes and 10 seconds/490 seconds if you're taking your time.

As you get fitter, or if you're already fit when you start the exercise routine, then the amount of rest-time taken between exercises can be dramatically reduced. It can easily be reduced by 50% or more. In fact, there's no reason why someone who performs this workout on a regular basis, shouldn't be able to reduce the amount of rest time between each exercise to between only 10 and 20 seconds. This makes it easily possible to perform the complete total-body exercise routine in as little as only 119 seconds, or 1 minute and 59 seconds.

Even with long rest periods factored-in, there is still a considerable amount of time which is saved by using the ISOfitness™ system, especially when compared to traditional methods of gym-based exercise. The realistic projections for how much time fitter people would save is astonishing. For example, let's take an advanced athlete, or a sports professional, who suddenly face an unavoidable time-crunch situation.

They can still benefit from a professional gym-level workout routine with the ISOfitness™ system. Even when exercising at the very highest levels of intensity, it still won't take long to complete a total-body workout. Furthermore, the ISOfitness™ workout can be performed almost anywhere relatively unobtrusively. So, the professional athlete can still get a high-level total-body workout no matter where they are, even while travelling as a passenger in a car, on a train, or on a plane. The result? The workout is not missed, and the time-crunch is resolved.

The Science

There are three basic types of resistance training. One type is isometric, which are exercises performed without any measurable movement of the limb becoming involved. The second type is isotonic exercise, which is all about movement. The third is isokinetic exercise, which is also about movement, however, with certain modifications to standard isotonic exercise applying to speed, velocity and force. Isokinetic exercises are not as commonly practised as regular isotonic exercises.

An exercise is isotonic when the tension remains the same, whilst the length of the muscle changes, such as when lifting and lowering a weight. There are two parts to an isotonic contraction, these are: concentric (lifting) and eccentric (lowering). In a concentric contraction, the muscle tension rises to meet the resistance, then remains the same as the muscle shortens. In the eccentric, the muscle lengthens due to the resistance being greater than the force the muscle is producing.

Isokinetic and isotonic contractions appear to be the same, however, they are technically very different. During exercise, an isotonic contraction will keep force at a constant, while velocity changes. An isokinetic contraction will keep velocity at a constant, while the force changes. In other words, no matter how much effort is applied the velocity remains fixed, however, the resistance experienced by the muscles through the limb's range of motion will change. Isokinetic exercises can be performed very effectively with an Iso-Bow®.

All three are excellent at building strength, and muscle size, as well as providing many other physical and health-related benefits. However, science has proven that one properly performed isometric exercise at only 2/3rds of an individual's overall maximum can deliver either similar or often better results, than the equivalent of up to 3 sets of 10 weight training repetitions. This is because when performed properly, and at the correct level of intensity, isometric exercise engages many more muscle fibres that can be achieved with regular weight training.

Comparison studies were carried out at the world-famous Max Plank Institute in Dortmund, Germany, over a 5-year period. The results of these experiments were published in the ground-breaking book: 'The Physiology of Strength,' by Dr Theodor Hettinger. They performed over 5,500 experiments on volunteers from all walks of life, from all age groups, on both sexes, and at every level of strength and fitness.

The results were revolutionary because they revealed the superiority of isometric exercise in building both strength and muscle much faster, and comparatively easier than isotonic exercise could. They also revealed something equally remarkable. This was that after performing only a single 7-second training stimulus (exercise) per day, the muscle being exercised was no longer responsive to further gains. The scientific data about this can be referenced on pages 28 to 31 of Dr Theodor Hettinger's book, "The Physiology of Strength."

Therefore, we don't typically recommend performing more than one isometric exercise in each position for each muscle group. The exception to this rule would be if a more advanced athlete wanted to develop a more constant strength-curve throughout the practical operational motion of a limb. This is because typically, the maximum strength gains during an isometric exercise are at the point which the isometric hold takes place, with additional benefits being gained in a strength-curve of as much as +20% and -20% of that initial point. Therefore, even an advanced athlete would probably only need to perform the isometric exercise at 2, or possibly 3 points, along the entire range of motion of the limb. Another exception would if an advanced or professional level athlete was employing a TRISOmetric™ exercises technique.

Another compelling research study revealed that the levels of muscle activation during repetitions of maximal weight training were between 89.7%, during the concentric contraction, or the lifting a weight, and 88.3% during the eccentric contraction, or the lowering of a weight. For practical purposes, about 89%. Scientific measurement also showed that during the lifting, or concentric, part of the exercise, the maximum intramuscular tension only lasted for between 0.25 and 0.5 seconds. Again, for practical purposes, about 1/3rd of a second. This is because traditional isotonic resistance exercises naturally involve movement, therefore, they also have aspects of velocity and acceleration to consider. Furthermore, "force" is only produced for a split second, to produce a maximal contraction of the muscle fibres.

However, the same research also clearly proved that the level of muscle activation during isometric exercise was as high as 95.2% and that it lasted for the entire 7 to 10 second period of each exercise. In addition to this, the muscle activation also lasted for a 7 to 10 second period of the isometric exercise, which is a huge increase over the 1/3rd of second muscular activation achieved during a single repetition of weight training. In practical terms, this means that if you're prepared to perform one daily isometric exercise for just 7 seconds, and at only 2/3rd's of your maximum effort, then it's possible to increase your strength by an average of up to 5% per week. If you can expect strength gains of an average of 5% per week in exchange for the expenditure of only 2/3rd's of your maximum effort, it's an excellent result!

As with all ISOfitness™ advanced isometric exercises, performing Iso-Bow® exercises will engage your body's natural Adaptive Response™ mechanism. If you always aim to perform the highest quality exercise, and at the highest level of intensity, you'll gain the maximum benefits possible in the shortest possible time. You can expect to become stronger, and fitter after each workout session. In theory, this means that for your next exercise session you will be a little stronger and fitter than you were for your previous session, which in turn means that you're able to put even more effort and intensity into your new exercise session than you did into the previous one. The cycle will then continue until you reach a physical plateau which is determined by your natural physical characteristics, capabilities, your age, and sex.

In respect of pure bodybuilding, even though isometric exercise is excellent at increasing muscle fibre density, size, and strength, pure bodybuilding requires an additional approach to deliver the maximum desired results. In pure bodybuilding, the quest isn't merely for strength, instead, it's all about muscle size, shape and aesthetics. Strength athletes would typically focus their training more on the prime mover muscles needed for strength related events. Bodybuilders will more widely spread the focus of their training to cover more of the muscle groups they want to develop. Isometric exercise will achieve both goals. However, the addition of the controlled pumping action of Dynamic Flexation™ will help to maximise both goals more efficiently.

Chapter 2: Strength at Only One Angle?

A common myth is that isometric contraction exercises only increases muscle strength at the specific angle at which the muscle and joint are exercised.

When talking about building strength in a broader range, rather than at a more specific point, one of the first things that should also be remembered is that during regular isotonic weight training, a constant-curve range of strength gain isn't achieved anyway.

Furthermore, this issue isn't as easily resolved using traditional isotonic resistance equipment as it is by performing isometric contraction exercises. The data clearly shows that in respect of isometric exercise, it's only partially true that there's only an increase in strength at the angle the contraction is engaged.

The scientific study performed by scientists Kitai and Sale called: "Specificity of Joint Angle in Isometric Training," concluded that strength gains were the greatest at the specific angle the training was performed.

It also concluded that there was a significant increase in strength along a much wider strength curve than previously thought. The study showed that there were increases in strength at the angles of +5 degrees, and -5 degrees to the isometric hold position.

More importantly, more extensive studies have subsequently found that with isometric contraction exercises, there is a much wider strength curve benefit than was first thought.

The later studies found that between 20% and 50% of strength-transfer occurs at the angles of +20 degrees, and -20 degrees to the isometric hold position.

It also concluded that there was a significant increase in strength along a much wider strength curve than previously thought. The study showed that there were increases in strength at the angles of +5 degrees, and -5 degrees to the isometric hold position.

This is huge, and it completely dispels all myths about any potential issues about this. The additional research also concluded that for those athletes who wanted to achieve the most complete and constant curve strength gain, it was comparatively easy to achieve with isometric contraction exercises, especially when compared to regular isotonic weight training.

To achieve the most complete and constant-curve strength gain possible, an advanced athlete would simply perform an isometric contraction exercise at two, three, or perhaps even more positions along the complete range of a joint/muscular range of motion.

To do this properly, it's worth briefly examining how this would work in practice, starting with a recap about biomechanics.

A normal, healthy limb has a certain Range of Motion, AKA: ROM. This is the arc through which the movement takes place at a joint, or series of joints. This ROM is technically called "Osteokinematic" motion.

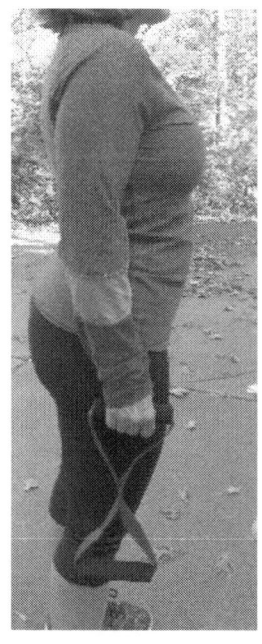
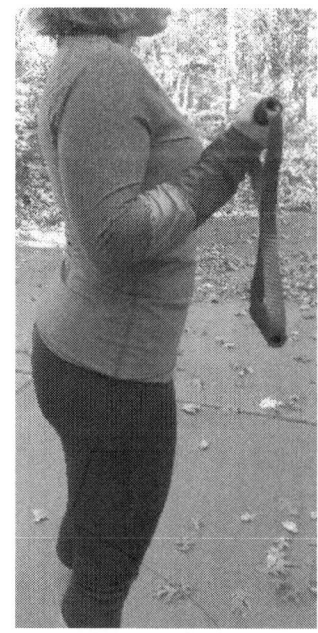

Zero Degrees   130 Degrees

Taking the biceps curl as an example, the range of motion for that movement in the pictures starts at zero when the hand is in the lower position and goes up to approximately 130 degrees in the upper position.

Next, if we assume that there's a strength-curve benefit of +20 degrees, and -20 degrees around the point at which an isometric contraction is performed, then we can calculate the approximate positions to perform the additional isometric contraction exercises.

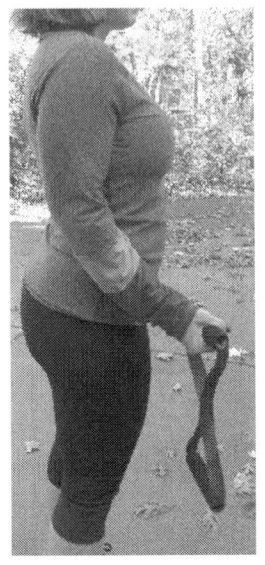

20 Degrees

The first position could be at approximately 20 degrees from the neutral starting point, because this would give a strength-curve benefit covering the first 40 degrees of the ROM.

The second position could be at approximately 50 degrees from the starting point, because this would safely overlap the first strength-curve arc from about the 30-degree point and extend up to about 70 degrees.

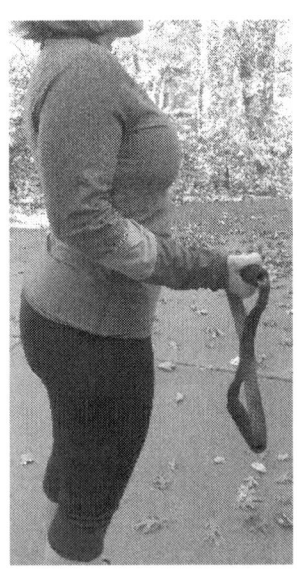

50 Degrees

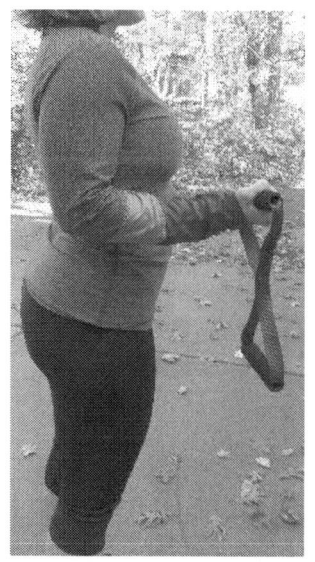

The last position could be at approximately 80 to 95 degrees from the starting point. This would then overlap the last, from the 60-degree point, and provide a strength-curve benefit across the higher end of the arc, getting closer towards the 130-degree maximum ROM of the limb.

80-95 Degrees

If necessary, a highly advanced athlete might also want to add an additional isometric contraction exercise at the starting point of the ROM of the limb. This would then strengthen the muscles when in the most mechanically disadvantaged position.

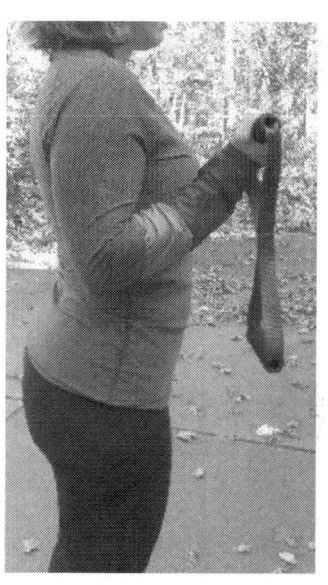

130 Degrees

Naturally, for those who are isometric enthusiasts like me, the information in this chapter is very interesting, however, does it relate to The Bullworker 90™ Course in some much deeper way?

Biceps, Supination, and Strong Arms

When most people think about the biceps muscles, they only think about flexing the biceps and elbow joint to create a classic bodybuilder biceps pose. However, there is a great deal more to the biceps muscles than this.

While flexing the arm in the way I've just described might be a primary function, another equally primary function is the action of twisting the forearm and hand, otherwise known as supination.

Supination starts with the hand in a neutral position, roughly parallel to the side of your upper thigh, and twisting it as it is being raised until your

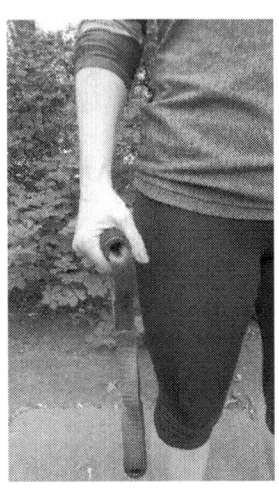

Neutral Position Front

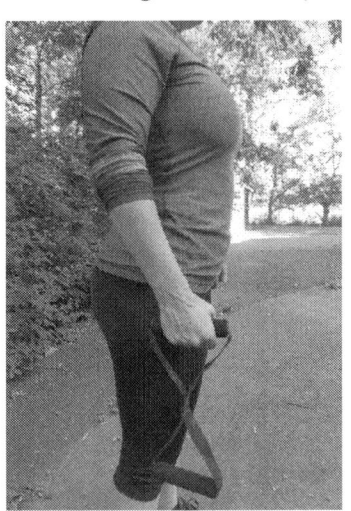

Neutral Position Side

palm is facing upwards at the top of the movement when the biceps are fully flexed.

The brachialis muscle is the primary mover of elbow flexion, and not the biceps brachii as most people think. This is because, even though the biceps brachii "show" muscle is seen flexed during a classic biceps pose, it is the brachialis which underlies it

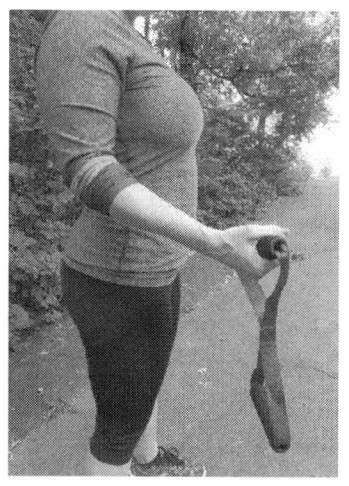

Mid Supination Side View

that generates about 50% more power than the biceps brachii. Therefore, supination is not only important to elbow rotation, but to overall upper arm strength. Therefore, to gain maximum benefit and strength when exercising your overall front upper arm, all component muscles and their actions must be taken into consideration.

A 'problem' with isometric exercise in this respect, when pitting only limb against limb, or against static immovable objects such as a wall, door or chair, is that it doesn't naturally allow the brachialis muscle to be exercised effectively.

The Iso-Bow®, and the Bow Extension kit offer an effective solution to this problem. These simple, yet highly effective devices allow a user to perform a wide range of exercises, either as a stand-alone device or in combination with other devices such as the Bullworker® and/or Steel Bow®. More importantly,

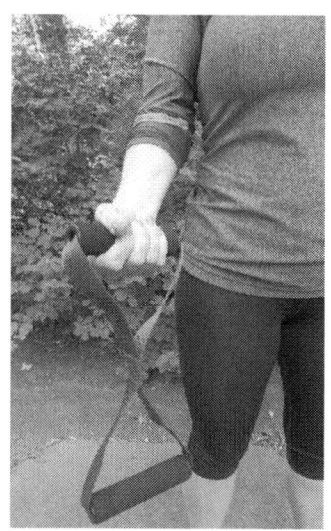

Mid Supination Front View

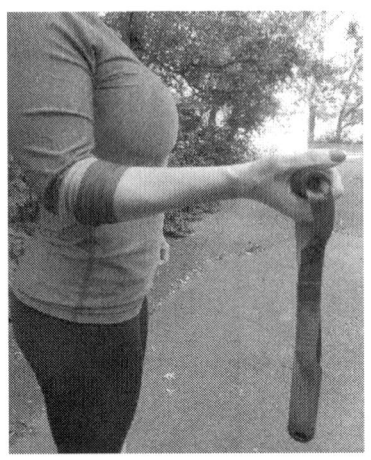

Full Supination Side View

they enable effective isometric and isotonic exercises to be performed in biomechanically correct ways.

Since the Iso-Bow® can be used to perform a wide range of barbell and dumbbell-like exercises either isometrically, or isotonically, this makes supination with the Iso-Bow® very easy. This makes it possible, and easy, to perform an isometric hold in both the neutral hand position, the semi-supinated hand position, and the fully supinated hand position.

Naturally, the same rules of exercise speed of motion, breathing, and correct biomechanical positioning apply to all concentric and eccentric actions. In respect of executing a biceps curl exercise in the best style possible, complete with supination, here are a few tips:

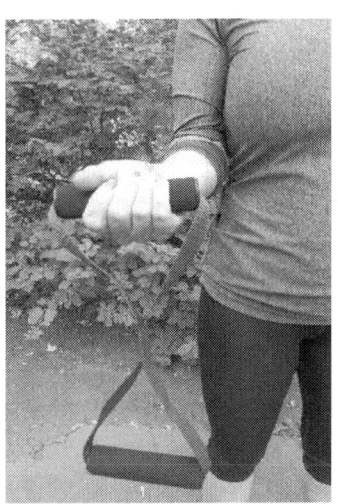

Full Supination Front View

- ⚠ As a rule, when performing a biceps curl, never allow your elbows to move forward, or kick-out to the side.
- ⚠ As with all curling exercises, never allow your wrist to bend backwards to fall out of alignment with the forearm because in this position, you're between 3 and 4 times weaker than if you hand and wrist was locked in correct biomechanical alignment.
- ⚠ In the starting position of any biceps exercise, always begin by firstly flex the triceps a little to ensure that you've fully lengthened the biceps, which will help to maximise the range of motion.
- ⚠ You can always adjust your gripping position on a hand grip to create and off-centre position because this will force your biceps to work even harder through supination.

Super-Slow Training

I believe that it's almost impossible to move too slowly during an exercise, however, it's easily possible to move too quickly. Super Slow is a form of strength training which was made popular by Ken Hutchins who worked at Nautilus and is based on an original concept by Dr Vincent Bocchicchio. He proposed that a single repetition of resistance training should take 10 seconds for the lifting phase, which is the concentric contraction where the muscles shorten. Pausing slightly to prevent momentum being generated. Then another 10 seconds for the lowering, or eccentric phase, where the muscles lengthen.

The super-slow concept incorporates extremely slow repetition speeds when compared to traditional resistance training protocols. In super-slow training, the emphasis is on minimizing momentum through minimal acceleration which improves muscular loading. Most research suggests that super-slow training yields better results in terms of strength gains and muscle growth than traditional resistance training methods.

The heart of the super-slow concept is based on the amount of tension a muscle develops. This is directly affected by the speed at which the muscle lengthens during the eccentric or lowering phase or shortens during the concentric or lifting phase of an exercise. The more tension that is generated, the more muscle fibres that are recruited. More importantly, the slower the myosin and actin filaments within the muscle fibres slide past each other, the more links that are formed between the filaments.

Therefore, using super-slow exercise speeds a maximum amount of tension is generated and a higher number of filament links are formed. In short, super-slow training activates more muscle fibres at an increased rate to maintain the force necessary to move the resistance provided. This is why it is a very efficient way to increase both strength and muscle size.

A typical super-slow workout would consist of one set of each exercise which is performed to the point of complete muscle fatigue/failure. Therefore, a 10-repetition exercise in such a routine would take between 200 and 250 seconds to perform in practice, with the overall workout session taking no longer than 30 minutes to complete. Since this is a high-intensity system, it requires greater rest time between workout sessions. Therefore, a workout frequency of twice each week is typically recommended.

One of the great advantages of super-slow training is in injury prevention. This is because in traditional resistance training, to make it more challenging more force is required through an increased resistance/weight being used. Therefore, the traditional method naturally increases the risk of injury. However, with super-slow training, you can make the exercise more challenging and engage more muscle fibres without increasing the force/weight.

A by-product of super-slow training is that it provides excellent cardiovascular benefits. This is because the heart is an involuntary muscle, therefore, it will always pump harder when there is more blood which needs pumping. Several studies have shown that super-slow training returns more blood to the heart than traditional aerobic training methods.

Chapter 3: The TRISOmetric™ Exercise Concept

I first developed the TRISOmetric™ exercise concept as a high-intensity method in the mid-1980's when I was training with 4-times World's Strongest Man Jon Pall Sigmarsson in Iceland. We were seeking to dramatically increase our training intensity without simply increasing the weight we were lifting and reducing our rest time between sets etc. If we could find a way to do this it would mean that we could more easily maintain a very high-intensity workout routine while travelling, when exercising at home, or back in the gym. We were successful in our quest, and the basis of my TRISOmetric™ exercise concept was born.

More importantly, as well as being able to be performed with traditional resistance equipment, or with no equipment whatsoever, other readily available commercial equipment can also be used. Therefore, the TRISOmetric™ exercise technique can be performed very easily with a Bullworker®, Steel Bow®, Iso-Bow®, and/or Iso-Gym®, or a combination of all of the above.

The TRISOmetric™ system combines 3 different angle maximum isometric exercises in combination with an isotonic exercise for the same muscle or muscle group. The three isometric exercises are performed first. Each exercise is performed in one of three positions in the range of motion of a limb or ROM. These are performed at maximum intensity in each position.

Each of the positions chosen will divide the range of motion of the limb roughly into three equal parts. This way a more even strength curve is developed for the muscle being exercised. This takes advantage of the strength gain overlap area of + and – 20% around the point of isometric exercise chosen.

It is very important that there should be no longer than 10 seconds of rest time between each isometric exercise. Once all three isometric exercises have been completed, then once again with a maximum rest time of 10 seconds, an appropriate isotonic exercise is used to exercise the same muscles or muscle group. This can be performed with either a Bullworker®, a Steel Bow®, an Iso-Bow®, and Iso-gym®, as freehand callisthenics or with weights/resistance machines. However, the method of performing this last exercise in the sequence should be in super-slow style. Each repetition should involve 10 seconds for the concentric or lifting phase where the muscles shorten, and another 10 seconds for the eccentric or lowering phase where the muscles lengthen.

If you perform each portion of each TRISOmetric™ exercise correctly, then you will find it extremely intense. I'd recommend that you do not attempt to repeat the exercise again and that you don't perform any other exercise for the same muscle/muscle group. If you perform the TRISOmetric™ exercise correctly you won't be able to, and, you won't want to do more. it's all about focus, intensity and the quality of what you do, and jot about the quantity.

During the experimental phase as I developed the TRISOmetric™ exercise concept, I concluded that it was better for the CNS, or Central Nervous System, to perform the isometric phases first. The data I gathered from several research papers clearly indicated that this made each isometric exercise more effective. Since one of the great advantages of isometric exercise is the efficiency factor, then this was foremost in my thoughts when I devised the TRISOmetric™ system.

The maximum 10 second rest period is just enough to allow the muscle being exercised to almost fully recover before the next exercise is applied. Naturally, this will place a high demand on the cardiovascular system of anyone performing this system. Therefore, if this is an issue, simply reduce the level of applied intensity during each isometric exercise accordingly. Eventually, your overall fitness level will increase to allow you to perform higher intensity exercises during each phase of the TRISOmetric™ exercise you're performing. Never be tempted to perform more sets, this is counter-productive. It should always be about aiming for maximum intensity during each exercise. If you're able to perform another set of an exercise, then you've not been applying maximum intensity to your previous one. Remember, it's inversely proportional. As the level of exercise intensity you apply increases, then the length of time that you are able to perform the exercise for decreases accordingly.

Initially, I also recommend that you perform the basic exercises for each body part. For example, you can perform either a power rack squat, wall squat, or an Iso-Bow® squat in 3 positions as isometric exercises. One could be while your thighs are parallel to the floor, the next position about 20 degrees higher, and the last position about 20 degrees higher again. With those completed, you could then perform a Bullworker® squat in super-slow exercise style, a power rack, or a freehand squat instead.

Another example would be to perform a combination of a Bullworker® and Steel Bow® chest press as an isometric exercise in three positions over the range of motion you have. After they have been completed, then aim to perform 10 isotonic repetitions in super-slow exercise style using either the Bullworker®, the Steel Bow or by performing push-ups. Once you have mastered achieving the 3 equal isometric exercise positions for each TRISOmetric™ exercise, then you have quite a wide selection of isotonic exercises to choose from to complete the exercise.

Chapter 4: Workout Intensity

"Intensity" is always going to be a relative term, and it's often completely misunderstood when it's used in relation to exercise. Basically, when it comes to exercising your muscles, the intensity is the % of your ability to move a resistance. Technically, an individual's highest possible level of intensity is when they reach a point of momentary failure after exerting themselves completely.

However, the important questions we need to try and find answers to are: "How hard is hard?" and "How intense is intense?" To some degree, both are very subjective things. Taking two people of roughly equal fitness, something that is intense to one person might be considered comparatively easy to the other.

"Hard" is also a relative term, and even 50lbs of resistance is impossibly hard if your strength is only at the level required to lift 49lbs. However, if you're able to lift a 100lbs as a maximum, then lifting 50lbs is going to be comparatively easy. Often, the only factors differentiating between people and the intensity level exerted, are going to be mental toughness, determination, and perception.

The human brain has a built-in mechanism which helps to protect the body and prevent it from performing physical activity to such a level that could cause serious damage, or even death. This is the mechanism that makes your brain tell you to stop exercising when it begins to get tough, and the feeling of wanting to stop exercising only increases as you continue to push yourself harder to do more. This is all despite the biological fact that you're physically capable of doing much more than is being suggested by the messages you're receiving from yourself.

Over time, the brain of people who exercise regularly, and especially to a high level of intensity, will naturally adjust and reposition this built-in safety margin. This means that the brain of an experienced high-level athlete doesn't "tell" them to stop an exercise until the level of intensity is much higher than it would be for a beginner.

Therefore, when it comes to exercise, how is it possible to subjectively quantify, and then impart appropriate levels of recommended intensity? This problem is made even more challenging when one considers the fact that accurately translating and subjectively assessing various levels of intensity will, to some degree, always be subjective to every individual.

If you really do train as hard as humanly possible, with near 100% maximum intensity, which involves super-strict form, training to complete failure, and beyond, then you simply can't train for a long period of time. It's just physiologically impossible. The physics and biology are very simple in this respect.

The intensity of your workout is directly proportional to the length of time that you're physically able to perform your workout. The harder and more intensely you exercise, then the shorter time that you'll be physically able to perform the exercise.

Make no mistake, performing a 7-second isometric exercise while exerting close to your personal 100% maximum physical capacity is completely and utterly exhausting, even for a professional athlete. What does all this mean when it comes to accurately communicate various levels of exercise intensity, especially when there's no professional coach or elaborate and expensive measuring equipment at hand?

The first and most obvious thing to remember is that research clearly shows that almost everyone will stop exercising long before they're in any danger of becoming seriously fatigued. Most people will *"think"* they're achieving a much higher level of intensity than they would do if they were only a little more mentally resilient.

This doesn't mean that people should suddenly begin pushing themselves beyond their physical limits, which would be a stupid thing to do. However, it does mean that most people who enjoy a higher than average level of mental resilience and determination, as well as being in physically good condition, can push themselves much harder than they might think. If anyone ever feels "genuine" strain or fatigue to the point of becoming injured, then they should stop exercising immediately.

Even without the aid of a professional coach to monitor, encourage you and measure your intensity and progress with specialist equipment, the tips we've outlined in this section will help you to get the most out every workout. It's also worth remembering that if you cheat, then the only person who really loses every time is "you."

Cardio, ISOfitness™, and Rest Time Between Exercises

If you keep the rest time between exercises brief enough, then the workout routine itself will give you an excellent cardiovascular workout, and this is what we recommend that you ultimately aim for.

If you're already very fit, then we'd recommend that instead of performing the optional cardio routine, and you simply put more effort and intensity into each isometric exercise. At the same time, aim to keep the rest time between those exercises as brief as possible.

This approach will help you work towards being able to perform each exercise so that it has an Ultra-High Intensity Ultra-Short Burst™ effect, which will greatly improve your overall fitness level, and boost your Base Metabolic Rate or BMR.

However, if you're not already fit, then to begin with you may wish to simply allow each isometric exercise to deliver all the cardio you need as you gradually build up your levels of fitness and endurance. Eventually, you'll soon increase your level of fitness to a point where you can begin to significantly, and steadily, reduce the rest time between each exercise to a minimum point that works best for you.

Once you've learned how to fully engage the muscles during each exercise with sufficient intensity, and at the same time you've learned how to breathe fully, deeply, and naturally throughout each exercise, while at the same time keeping the rest time between exercises to a minimum, then this combination will have an excellent and beneficial cardiovascular effect.

Ultra-High Intensity, Ultra-Short Burst™

Short bursts of high-intensity exercise are extremely effective at breaking down the body's stored reserves of glucose in the muscles, which is called glycogen. When these reserves of glycogen are rapidly depleted due to the high-intensity bursts of exercise, it creates room for the glucose in your blood to replace it and be stored instead. In short, it removes some of the sugar circulating in your bloodstream, which in turn has both overall health and weight loss benefits.

Research carried out by Professor Jamie Timmons of Nottingham University in England conducted a four-year detailed scientific study with over 1000 test subjects about the efficacy of Ultra-High Intensity Ultra-Short Burst™ exercise in comparison with other types of exercise. Unsurprisingly, they found that the key to gaining the greatest benefits from exercise was based on extremely short high-intensity exercise sessions, and not in lengthy, prolonged workouts.

However, their research also concluded something quite remarkable which is that as little as 3 minutes per week of ultra-high intensity exercise, performed in extremely short bursts of only 10 seconds each, is all that's needed to significantly boost a person's Base Metabolic Rate (BMR), dramatically improve cardiovascular efficiency, improve their overall health, and get them into great shape too.

This 10-second "magic" number for a basic Ultra-High Intensity Ultra-Short Burst™ exercise routine is a perfect length of exercise time. This is because it coincides perfectly with the 7 seconds of time needed to perform a practical high-intensity isometric exercise, together with the few extra seconds of exercise which are always needed to properly engage, and then disengage the muscles and joints.

This means that when performed at a very high level of intensity, isometric exercises have a similar effect to a basic Ultra-High Intensity Ultra-Short Burst™ exercise routine. Beyond this Ultra-High Intensity Ultra-Short Burst™ advanced isometric exercise effect, advanced and professional athletes can then factor in the amount of rest time taken between exercises.

According to the highly acclaimed and pioneering sports scientist, Arthur Jones, the man who invented the famous Nautilus system, muscle recovery has a half-life which occurs every 3 seconds after an exercise has been stopped. This means that in as little as 9 seconds of rest time you're ready to begin your next exercise. Naturally, 9 seconds is a very brief period, and after performing a high-intensity exercise your heart and lungs will be working exceptionally hard.

Aiming for a consistent 9 second rest time target between each exercise is going to be incredibly challenging, and it's something which is only possible for people who are already exceptionally fit, advanced, semi-pro, and professional athletes. When beginning exercises for the first time, most people will take a much longer rest period between exercises, especially if they're performed at an average of approximately 2/3rds of someone's personal maximum capacity.

We'd suggest that you don't rush any of this and that only as you gradually improve your levels of fitness, then you can also aim to gradually reduce the amount of rest time taken between exercises. We'd always recommend that you always practice maximum caution in all things, especially when it comes to pushing yourself to new, higher limits in your workout routine.

Always do this with safety in mind, take your age and physical ability into consideration, and never to push yourself beyond your personal safe limits. This would be the safest, and most efficient way to work towards the goal of performing each exercise in your workout routine as an Ultra-High Intensity Ultra-Short Burst™ exercise, followed by only a maximum of 9 to 10 seconds of rest time between each exercise. At this point, you'll be giving yourself one of the most effective cardiovascular workouts possible, while you'll also be performing the most efficient strength and muscle building exercises possible.

Strength, Stamina, Endurance, and Resilience

It is important to understand the difference between strength, stamina, and endurance, because once understood, you'll then be able to devise the most suitable workout routines according to your body type.

Muscular strength is possibly best understood as being a muscle's capacity to exert force against resistance, or weight. This is comparatively easy to measure because your ability to lift a given amount of weight for a single repetition is a good measure of your strength.

Stamina is the length of time at which a muscle, or group of muscles, can perform at or near your maximum capacity. For example, the number of squats you can perform with a given weight which is 90% of your maximum would be a measure of your stamina or the distance which you can carry a similarly heavy object such as an anvil.

Endurance is all about time, and your ability to perform a certain muscular action for a prolonged period regardless of the capacity at which you're working.

Resilience is all about your ability to recover from whatever stresses and demands are placed upon your muscles. However, resilience is mostly all about your state of mind, your mental toughness and ability to endure, perform and deliver under pressure, and to recover quickly emotionally.

The muscular composition of your body will always determine how well you will perform at certain sports. The amount of slow twitch muscle fibres you possess will determine how well you perform at endurance related events, and both type A and type B fast twitch muscle fibres are all about explosive power and your ability to maintain it.

If you possess mostly slow twitch fibres, then you're naturally better suited to endurance sports. Alternatively, if you possess mostly fast twitch muscle fibres, then you're a natural weightlifter.

It's important to note, that no matter what your natural predisposition might be in this respect, with the correct training regimen, it is still possible to significantly increase your abilities in your naturally weaker opposing areas of speciality.

Rest and Recovery

For those who have already read about this subject in "The 70 Second Difference™" book, they will know that rest and recovery after intense exercise is essential. This is because your body, and immune system, must be given sufficient time to recuperate properly.

If it's your intention to significantly increase your muscle size and strength, then it's always worth remembering that your muscles don't grow during your workout. The workout phase is the stimulus, and the real growth process begins after your workout is over, during the recovery period.

Exercising too often will prevent complete recovery from taking place, and it will eventually deplete your muscle tissue and have the complete opposite effect to what you wish to achieve.

When calculating your ideal recovery period many things must be taken into consideration including your age, your current health and fitness level, the quantity of exercise taken, and most importantly the intensity of the exercise which has been performed.

Some people will need a recovery period of between 24 and 48 hours, and for others, the recovery period may be as brief as between 12 and 24 hours. However, as a rule, the recovery period will incrementally increase as the intensity of the exercises increases towards an individual's 100% potential maximum capacity.

Sports scientist J. Atha's research revealed something remarkable. This was that when performing isometric contraction exercises at 2/3rd's of an individual's maximum capacity, the average person could safely perform an exercise like this daily, without overtraining.

Standard isometric exercises can be safely performed daily, by almost anyone, of almost any age, and in almost any physical condition as a means of strength development, body shaping, and even for bodybuilding.

For other workouts that are more intense, then we recommend a full rest day between workouts due to the higher demands being placed upon the Central Nervous System (CNS).

There are several other factors which affect post-exercise recovery. These include a balanced and properly executed stretching routine and getting enough quality sleep. While you sleep, your body releases certain hormones which help you to repair and rebuild damaged tissue, and which will directly help your muscles to grow.

Post-exercise high-quality nutrition will help your body to repair itself faster, decrease your recovery time, and will help to generally maximise the benefits gained from the exercise.

Studies indicate that there is a 30 to 60-minute time-window after exercise when you need to eat, and after which, your body begins to draw upon itself to repair and recover from your exercise session.

Drinking enough water is also one of the most important factors in your recovery, as well as for your overall health because your muscles are mostly composed of water.

Dynamic Flexation™

We'll recap and briefly summarise the Dynamic Flexation™ technique as laid out in "The 70 Second Difference™" book. Even for a beginner, we would always recommend that to some degree everyone employs a form of Dynamic Flexation™.

This will help to ensure that all muscles, tendons, ligaments, joints, and spine become naturally and properly engaged in the correct isometric exercise position, which will usually be helped by taking a correct hand grip, fist clench, or foot position.

You should always ensure that you perform each exercise in the correct biomechanical position to gain maximum benefit from each exercise. When you assume the correct position, to begin with, you should apply almost no tension whatsoever.

Instead, you should "feel" your way into ensuring that you're in the correct position *before* beginning to apply tension to the exercise. Once you're in the correct position, perhaps the worst thing to do would be to suddenly apply maximum tension and at the same time hold your breath. This is completely wrong. Instead, remember to always breathe naturally as you gradually engage your muscles into the exercise.

Our personal preference is to apply the tension gradually through Dynamic Flexation™, over a period of up to 3 or even 4 seconds. This is before beginning to count the required 7-second exercise hold of the isometric contraction. During the exercise, be sure to breathe naturally and deeply.

We prefer using each full breath in and out as a method of counting more accurately the number of seconds each exercise is performed, with one breath in and out representing one second. Similarly, at the end of an exercise, we don't recommend that it be ended abruptly. Instead, we prefer to reverse the Dynamic Flexation™ technique, and to gradually relax and slightly move each muscle and joint as you do so.

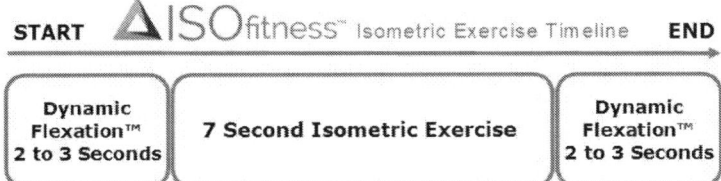

Dynamic Flexation™ is a concept which embraces the broader principles of motor unit recruitment, and "Henneman's Size Principle," to increase the contractile strength of a muscle. Elwood Henneman's principle stated that, under load, the motor units in a muscle are engaged according to their magnitude of force output, from the smallest to the largest, and in task-appropriate order.

This means that the slow-twitch, low-force, fatigue-resistant muscle fibres are activated before any fast-twitch, high-force muscle fibres are engaged which are less fatigue-resistant. Since the body works in this way, it enables precise, finely controlled force to be delivered at all levels of output. This also means that when exercising, or when performing tasks in daily life, the fatigue which is experienced as a result will be always be minimised, and proportional to the sequential engagement of the most appropriate muscle fibres.

What is ISOfitness™ and TWiEA™?

The ISOfitness™ exercise system is the name we use to cover all the exercises we write about and teach. The core of the ISOfitness™ exercise system is based solidly on the original, proven isometric science. However, the ISOfitness™ system is much more than that alone. It incorporates the new, advanced isometric exercise discoveries and techniques including, Dynamic Flexation™, Super-Slow Isotonic Flexation™, and the newly proven science of USB-UHT™ (Ultra Short Burst – Ultra High Intensity) exercises. The ISOFitness™ exercise system also includes our own resultant hybrid TRISOmetric™ exercise system.

The 70 Second Difference™ Book

"The 70 Second Difference™" book covers all aspects of the ISOfitness™ exercise system. It particularly focusses on more of the science and practical application of the major forms of isometric exercises. This includes the science of strength, muscle growth, weight-loss, nutrition, and other important things related to fitness, strength training, bodybuilding, and body shaping. It also contains a comprehensive 7 exercise workout routine that will exercise all the main muscles of the body in only 70 seconds of consecutive exercise time. There is even a choice of workout sessions suitable for the beginner, intermediary, and more advanced athlete.

"The 70 Second Difference™" book is designed to be the foundation base-reference guide which will support all the books we produce including this one. In taking this approach, it means that we won't be repeating ourselves, or at least when we do it will be kept to a minimum, and only because we believe that we need to reinforce some extremely important point/s.

TWiEA™ Resources.

All ISOfitness™ online resources have now been absorbed into The World Isometric Exercise Association, or TWiEA™ for short (www.TWiEA.com). The World Isometric Exercise Association, TWiEA™, is the global governing body for all types of isometric exercise. TWiEA™'s mission is to help set and maintain standards of excellence in teaching and promoting all types of isometric exercise

It was formed because most exercise coaches and gyms don't promote and recommend isometric exercises is because of the following: A) they lack training/real knowledge to teach isometrics properly, B) self-serving commercial interests mean that recommending isometric exercise could deeply impact their training/membership fees.

it's ironic that the exercise systems that most exercise professionals recommend to their clients are the systems that take the most time to perform. Therefore, they're actually the exercise systems that people will most likely stop using!

In the global quest to improve health and fitness by encouraging people to exercise regularly using traditional time-consuming methods, coaches and personal trainers who do this are actually compounding matters to become part of the overall problem. Since lack of time is typically the #1 reason restricting and/or preventing people from getting the high-level workout they need, coaches should be recommending real-life time-efficient exercise solutions that busy people can follow.

TWiEA™'s mission is to ensure that scientifically proven time-efficient isometric exercise techniques are taught to clients as part of an integrated overall approach to the total-body exercise solutions provided by fitness professionals. This creates a much higher probability that clients who are busy people, and who often face real-life time-crunches, can still maintain a regular highly effective exercise program.

The fact is that isometric exercise is every bit as effective, and frequently more effective, at building muscle and strength as other more traditional forms of resistance training. It is also a time-saving and money-saving exercise solution that almost anyone can perform, even without equipment.

Chapter 5: The Iso-Bow® and Other Devices

A common question we're asked is: "is it necessary to use the Iso-Bow® to perform an effective isometric or self-resisted workout?"
This is a very good question. No, it's not necessary to use an Iso-Bow®, but we believe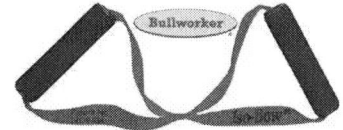
that it is better if you do, and there are several reasons why.

Firstly, it's all about the science and safety of biomechanics. A stable line of biomechanical progression all begins with a correctly positioned grip, a firm grip, and the progression in continuing that stability through correctly aligned joints and limbs while you perform the exercise.

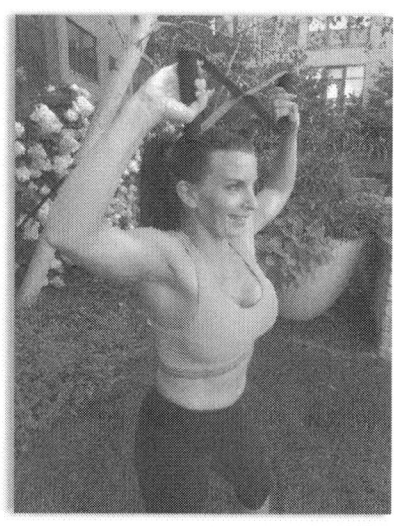
The same is true in isometric exercise because it all begins with a stable line of biomechanical progression. This starts with either a properly clenched hand or fist and continuing that stability through correctly aligned joints and limbs to perform the isometric hold.

This is just one reason why we fully recommend and endorse the Iso-Bow® because it makes this whole process much easier. It has a well-designed and comfortable nonslip hand grip, which allows you to execute a firm, stable hand grip position to begin creating a stable line of biomechanical progression.

The Iso-Bow® is a product we fully endorse and highly recommend. It's inexpensive, high quality, and it 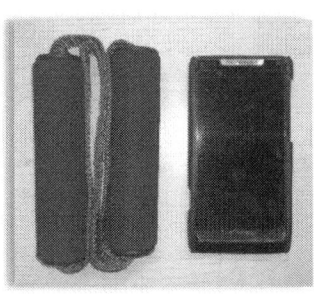 works exceptionally well. An amazing Iso-Bow® costs "pennies" in comparison to other exercise devices, and even a pair of them can easily fit into your pocket, they never need adjusting, they can deliver a total-body workout at the perfect level of intensity for either a complete unfit beginner or an advanced athlete!

If you've already read "The 70 Second Difference™" book, then you'll also know that we're not even endorsing our own product. We're simply endorsing a product which we believe will be the best investment you'll ever make if you want to get fit, strong, and in the best shape of your life. The company that makes the Iso-Bow® is Hughes Marketing LLC, and they also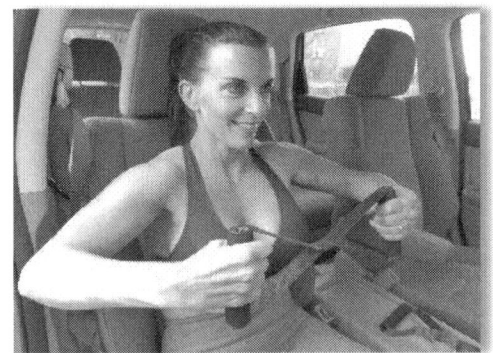

produce a small range of other highly effective exercise products, which all deliver excellent results at a fair price.

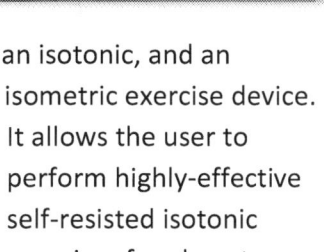

The Iso-Bow® is versatile too, and it can be used with equal effectiveness as both an isotonic, and an isometric exercise device. It allows the user to perform highly-effective self-resisted isotonic exercises for almost every muscle group.

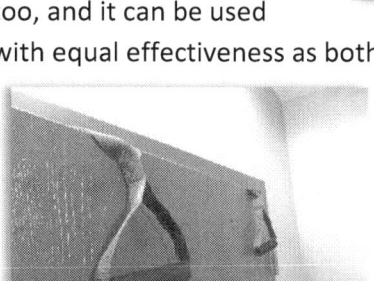

A pair of Iso-Bows® can even be used as a great doorway pull-up device, which can even fold up and slip right into your pocket when you're done. Try doing that with a regular, clumsy steel doorway pull-up bar!

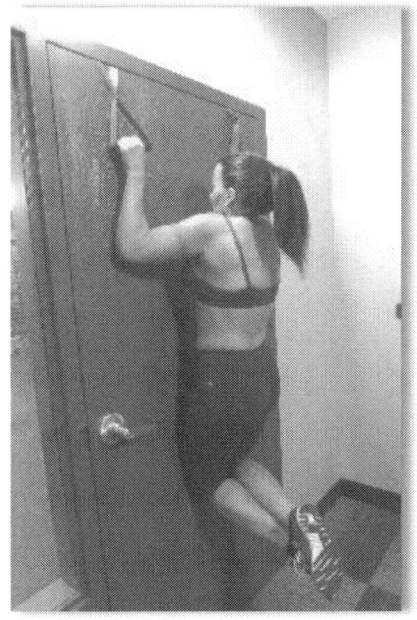

The Iso-Bow® is naturally a first-class isometric exercise device, and it allows a very wide range of exercises to be performed that work almost every muscle group of the body. It also allows the effective execution of more advanced techniques to be performed within the ISOfitness™ system.

Since the Iso-Bow® is so inexpensive, well designed, well-constructed, and extremely useful in ways we haven't even begun to describe here in this book, it's not so much a recommendation for you to get a pair, rather an instruction for you to do so. We believe that you'll soon see why these inexpensive devices are what we believe to be the finest, most versatile, and most powerful of all exercise devices which have ever been invented!

That's a bold statement, but it's made from our heart, and it's delivered with our most sincere belief in the product and how you will benefit from owning a pair, and in using them correctly. Don't forget, we don't make this product, we simply believe in it to that degree of commitment.

Securing the Iso-Bow® With Your Feet

When performing leg exercises such as squats and lunges, as well as lower back and glute exercises such as deadlift, it becomes necessary to properly secure the Iso-Bow® using your feet.

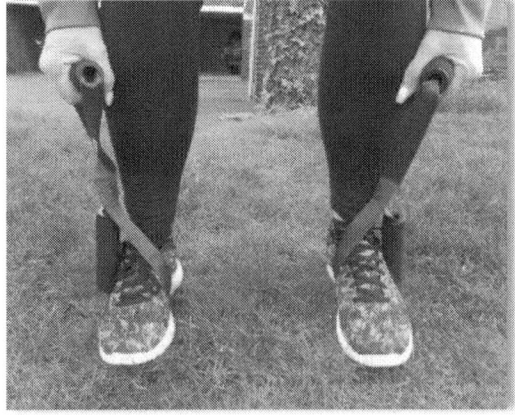

There are several ways in which the Iso-Bow® can be secured using your feet, and your personal preference of how you do this will depend upon many factors such

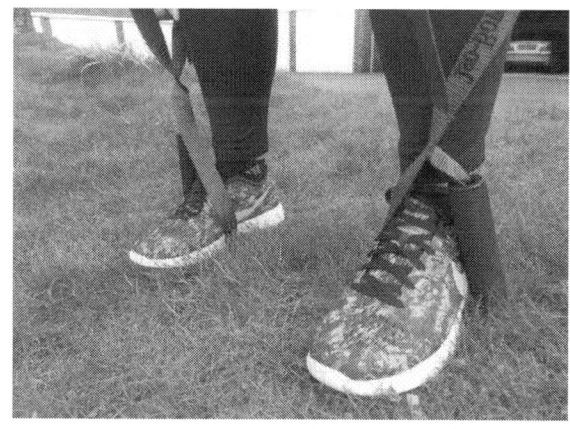

as your foot size, your choice of footwear, and ease of operation.

You can secure the Iso-Bow® with your foot inside one of the handles. You do this by adjusting the handgrip to

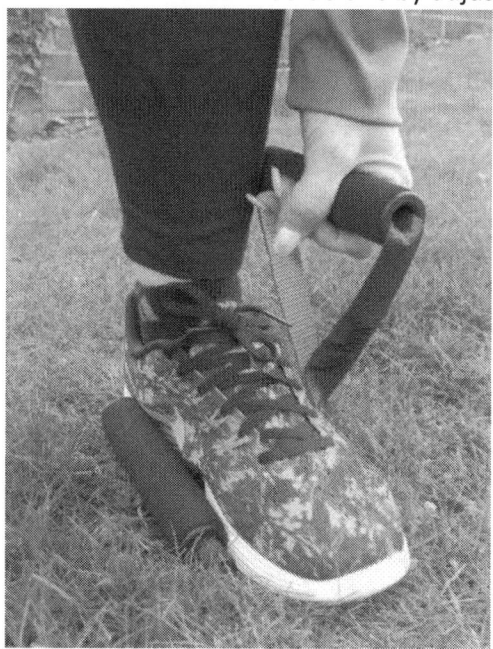

one side, usually the outer side of the foot, and then place your feet inside the loop like a stirrup.

Another method is to place the Iso-Bow® flat on the floor and then stand on one side of the straps so that the handle of the same side sits flush to your inner foot. In this position, it will be your bodyweight combined with the handle pressing against the inner side of your foot which enables you to pull safely and securely.

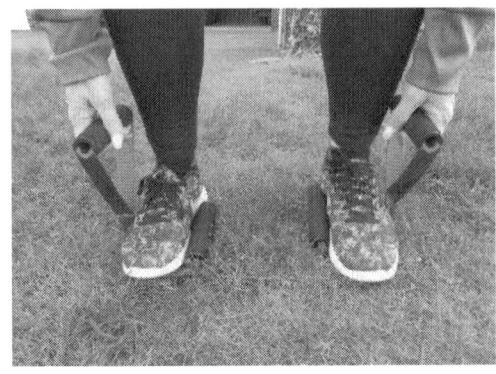

The final method is to simply place each foot through one end of an Iso-Bow®, stepping onto the foam hand grip as you do so. This method offers slightly less stability than the other two methods. However, if the foot can be pushed far enough through the loop of the Iso-Bow® handle,

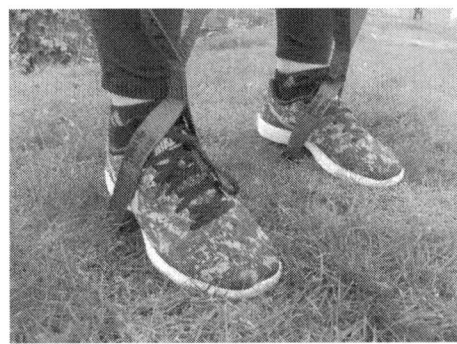

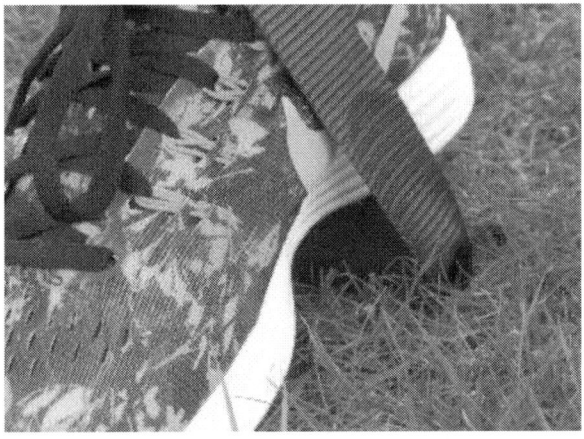

then the handle will slightly raise the level of your heel making it easier for some people to squat or lunge.

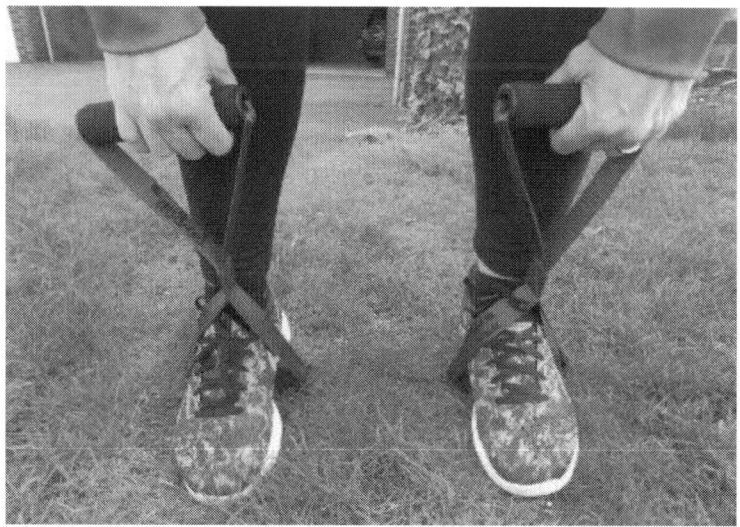

Naturally, safety is always a top priority so whichever method you ultimately choose to use, you should always make sure that when securing the Iso-Bow® with your feet that there is never any chance of it slipping in any way while you exercise.

The Bow Extension®

The Bow Extension® is a set of straps which are basically the handle of an Iso-Bow® at each end of a much longer intermediary strap. The exact length of each Bow

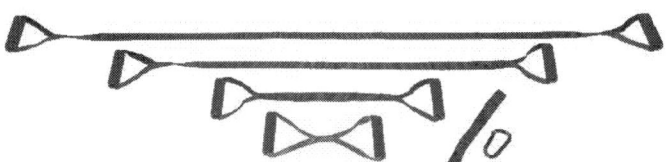

Extension® strap varies, and when combined as a set they are excellent straps which enable a wide range of advanced isometric exercises to be performed.

The Bow Extension® is also designed to be used to extend itself, the Iso-Bow®, or the range of motion in which the Bullworker® and/or Steel Bow® is used in various exercises.

Bow Extension

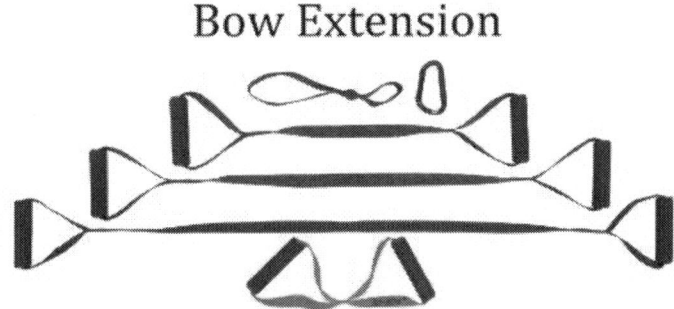

Extending the Iso-Bow® and Bow Extension®

A pair of Iso-Bows® or any combination of Bow Extension® straps can be interlocked so that it effectively increases the length of a single Iso-Bow® by somewhere between 50% and 75%. The same technique can be used to dramatically increase the length of the Bow Extension® straps. This can either be in combination with themselves, or with one or more Iso-Bows®.

This is achieved by looping one handle through the other, and then back through itself to form a secure attachment. Always keep the webbing flat where at all possible and ensure that the handles of each strap sit evenly and flush against each other.

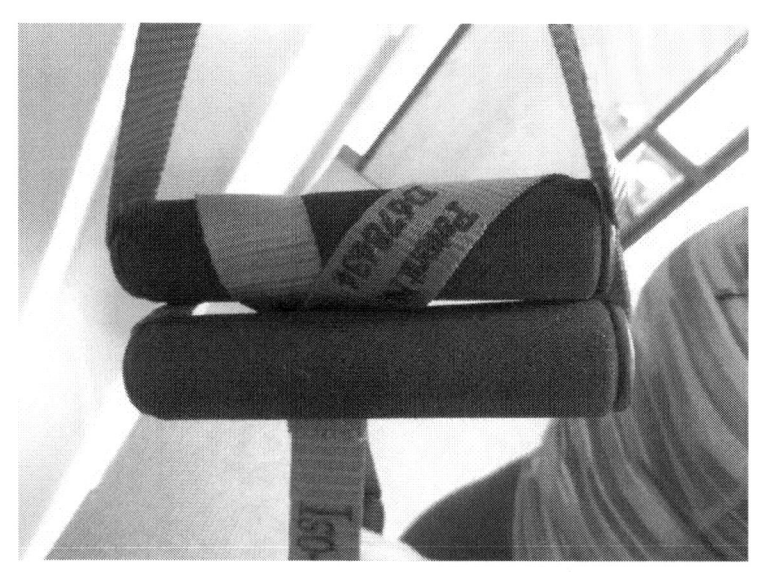
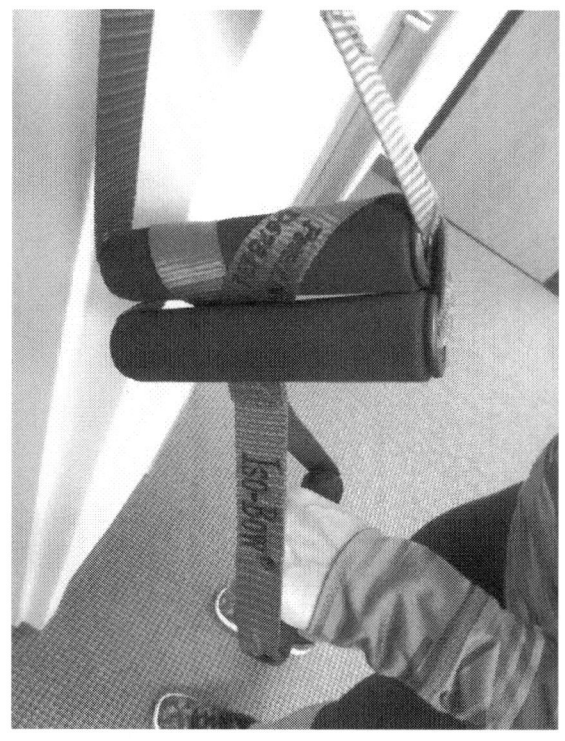

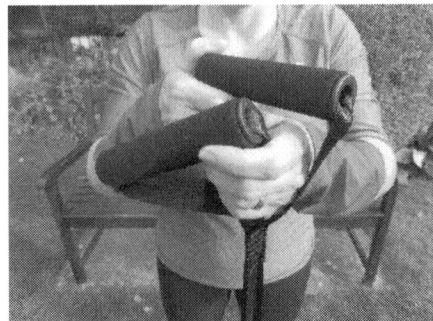

Place one handle through the loop of another handle.

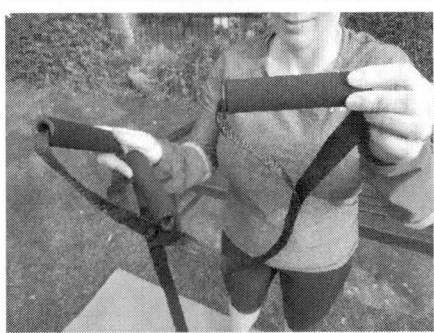

Pull the handle right through.

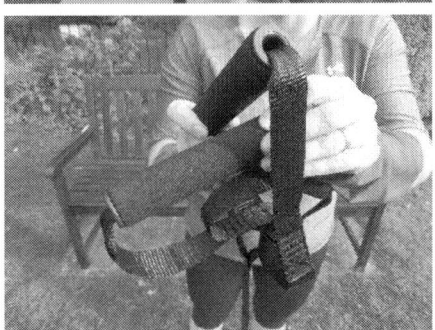

Then loop the other handle back through the first handle to form a secure loop.

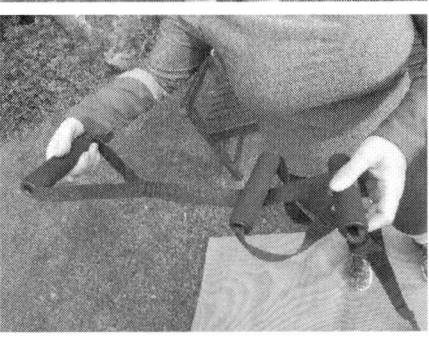

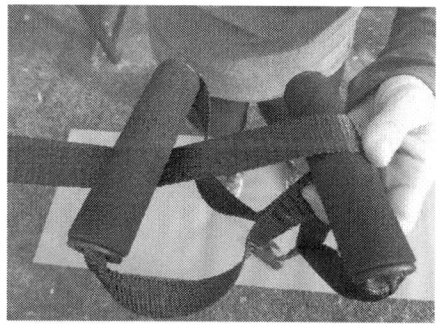

Ensure that the two handles and straps are not tangled.

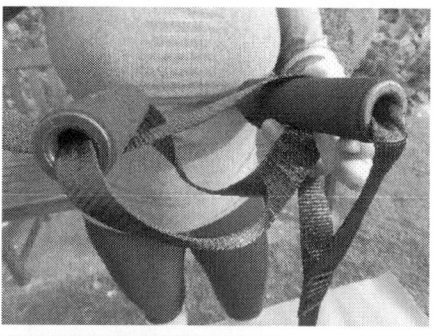

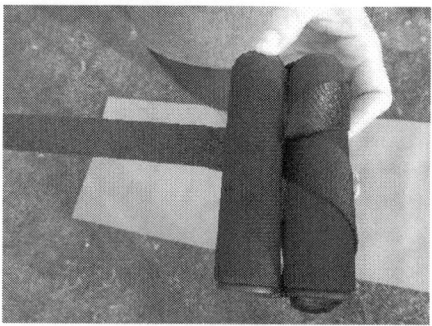

When the straps and handles are pulled tight, make sure that both handles sit neatly alongside each other.

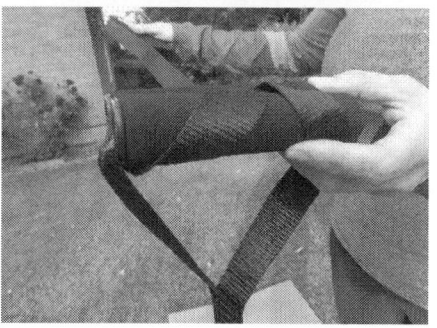

The Iso-gym®

The Iso-Gym®, depending on the model, is a self-resisted and bodyweight suspension exercise device. The length of Iso-Gym® strap can be adjusted, or specific length straps can be used to perform various exercises.

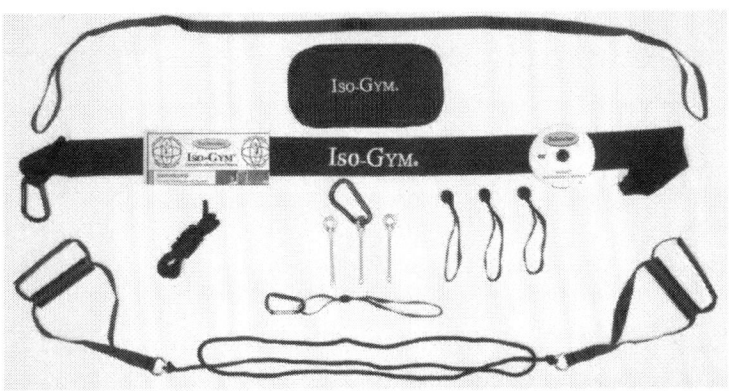

The Bullworker®

The Bullworker® is an exercise device which allows the user to perform either isometric exercises, or isotonic exercises, or a combination of the two. It is a proven and reliable device that has been used and endorsed by multiple World champions for several decades.

These include Muhammad Ali, Dave Prowse and Bruce Lee. The Bullworker has sold over 10 million units since it was first launched, and the modern device continues to be a best-seller.

It is approximately 36 inches long and can be used either as a stand-alone device or as a complete home gym when in combination with the Steel Bow®, the Iso-Bow®, the Bow Extension® and Iso-Gym®. It has two interchangeable springs with different levels of resistance.

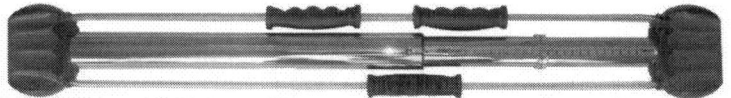

The Steel Bow®

The Steel Bow® is about 20 inches long and is basically a shorter version for the full-size Bullworker® Classic model. The Steel Bow® comes with 3 interchangeable springs of 3 different resistance levels.

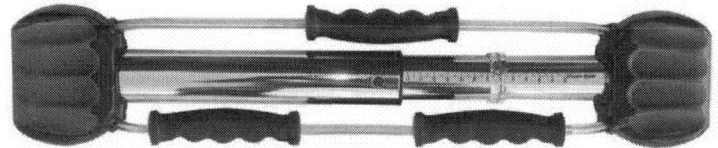

Other Equipment and Techniques

Many isometric exercises can be performed without an Iso-Bow®, Bow Extension®, Iso-Gym®, Bullworker® or Steel Bow®, using any or all of these devices makes it very much easier. They also allow certain exercises to be performed that would be either challenging or impossible without them.

Most, or all, of these devices can be used to perform isotonic exercises as well as isometric ones. This means that you have a much wider choice of exercises to choose from for the super-slow isotonic phase of each TRISOmetric® exercise. When these devices are combined with freehand callisthenics and tradition gym equipment it makes a powerful all-around combination.

Chapter 6: Things to Remember Before You Begin...

- ▲ The first and perhaps the most important thing to remember is: **NEVER HOLD YOUR BREATH AT ANY TIME, AND EACH DEEP BREATH WILL COUNT THE NUMBER OF SECONDS IN EACH EXERCISE**.
- ▲ Breathing in and out naturally during all isometric exercises will also help you count the number of elapsed seconds much more accurately.
- ▲ We recommend that you read the instructions about each workout routine and exercise carefully. You can also watch the associated videos on the ISOfitness™ website.
- ▲ Weight loss/fat loss will ONLY occur when ISOfitness™ exercises, or ANY other exercise plan, is used in conjunction with a calorie-controlled diet.
- ▲ It's critically important to completely focus your mind on the exercise being performed, and in addition to this, to fully envision the muscle growing and getting stronger.
- ▲ Always consult a professional coach to devise a detailed stretching routine, this will ensure that you're stretching the areas effectively rather than risking injury. Always ensure that a stable line of biomechanical progression is achieved before engaging in and performing any exercise.
- ▲ Warming-up, stretching, and cooling down are three of the most overlooked, yet essential elements to exercise, and we cannot stress their importance strongly enough. During ANY form of physical exercise, including isometrics, if you apply

too much intensity too soon, then you may inadvertently strain a muscle. Isometric exercise is particularly intense, and a single isometric exercise engages a great many more muscle fibres than even high-intensity weight training, and isometrics engages the muscle fibres at a much higher level too.

Therefore, for safety's sake, we're adamant that you should always gradually and progressively engage your muscles into ANY isometric exercise, and according to what we call The ISOfitness Exercise Timeline™.

The main benefit to properly warming up for several minutes before a workout is injury prevention, and to increase your heart rate and the circulation to your muscles, ligaments and tendons. It's important to remember that warming-up and stretching are two different concepts, and stretching isn't a good warm-up. This is because stretching will put the muscle in an un-contracted position and weaken it. Stretching is always best performed after a workout has been completed, together with a proper cool-down.

In addition to properly warming-up, always perform a gentle "flex and stretch" of the muscles and joints which are about to be exercised. For example, squatting down fully to flex the thighs and loosen the knees is always a good idea before performing any leg exercises. Dynamic

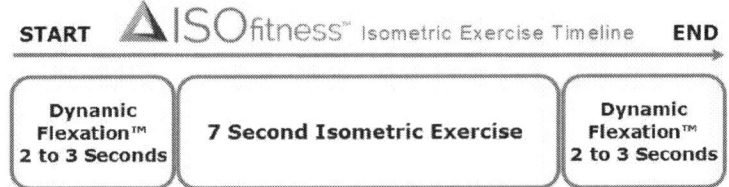

Flexation™ should always be used with every ISOfitness™ style isometric exercise. Here's a diagram which explains the workflow visually.

ISOfitness™ style isometric exercises are deceptively powerful. Even when engaging in what may feel like only moderate intensity exercise, you're probably still engaging and contracting a great many more muscle fibres than you would in a similar isotonic exercise. Therefore, if you're in any doubt whatsoever, then always perform the exercise with a little less intensity. In addition to a proper warm-up, the Dynamic Flexation™, performed in conjunction with the isometric exercise, will help to ensure greater blood supply to the muscles and surrounding tissue.

ALL ISOfitness exercises and workout plans work equally well for men AND women. BOTH sexes can build great strength, solid muscle, body build, or simply get into great shape if they wish, each according to their natural potential.

Just because Helen Renée usually demonstrates the exercises in our printed products, stills pictures, and in the videos on the members-side of the ISOfitness™ website, it doesn't mean that the exercises and products are only for women. They're NOT! The science, the exercises, the techniques, and the workout routines, all work equally well for both sexes at every level, from a complete beginner right up to a sports professional, bodybuilder, and strength athlete. Men who think this way, then get over any silly notion about this now! That's 'dinosaur' thinking!

Please read, review, and ensure that you've fully complied with all recommendations in the section entitled: *'Important General Safety and Health Guidelines,'* and only start ISOfitness™ exercises with the full approval of your physician.

Important Notes About Exercise Equipment Choices

We have deliberately chosen to demonstrate the isometric phase of each TRISOmetric exercise with either an Iso-Bow®, Bow Extension®, Iso-Gym®, Bullworker® or Steel Bow®. This is because they are specifically designed for this purpose and they work exceptionally well for isometric exercise purposes. Similarly, we have chosen either one of the aforementioned exercise devices or a freehand callisthenic exercise for the isotonic phase for the same reasons. You can choose whatever device you prefer to use for this phase, including resistance machines and weights.

However, if you perform the isometric exercises in the first phase of a TRISOmetric™ exercise properly, and with a maximum of only 10 seconds of rest time between exercises, then you will be extremely pre-exhausted. This means that you'll be performing the isotonic phase of your TRISOmetric™ exercise after a maximum of only another 10 seconds of rest time. Therefore, even with the best will in the world, you still won't be able to lift a heavy weight or apply much resistance to any type of exercise you choose. Since the last phase of your TRISOmetric™ exercise is a super-slow set of 10 repetitions, with the lifting phase taking 10 seconds per single repletion, and the lowering phase the same, your muscles will be crying out for mercy. In short, if you do your TRISOmetric™ exercise properly, then even a very strong person will only be able to use light weights.

It's important NOT TO CHEAT by speeding up the repetitions just to enable you to lift more weight. This will be totally counterproductive. So, take your ego out of the equation, and accept the fact that you'll probably only be able to lift about ¼ (or less) of what you'd normally lift, or perform a fraction of the repetitions when performing push-ups and squats, etc. you may even need to perform assisted repetitions which as push-ups from the knees instead of your feet. If that's all you can do, then accept it and get over it. Remember, this is all about growing muscle and strength, and it's not a competition to see what you can lift every time you exercise.

The exercises in the next chapter are merely suggestions. As are the number of exercise positions demonstrated. You may wish to substitute some of your own which you might prefer. The choice is yours, the important thing to remember is that an exercise becomes TRISOmetric® when any isometric hold is performed in three positions BEFORE a final isotonic exercise is performed using the super-slow technique.

About the Exercise Model

Helen Renée is the model in the section describing the exercises and how to perform them. Helen is a contest-winning bodybuilder and Bikini Fitness Competitor who exercises religiously every day, no matter where she is or where she's travelling to. Helen is particularly strong with the exceptional power-to-weight ratio one would expect from a former gymnast. She is also an isometric exercise expert instructor and instructor-trainer for TWiEA™ The World Isometric Exercise Association.   HelenRenee.com

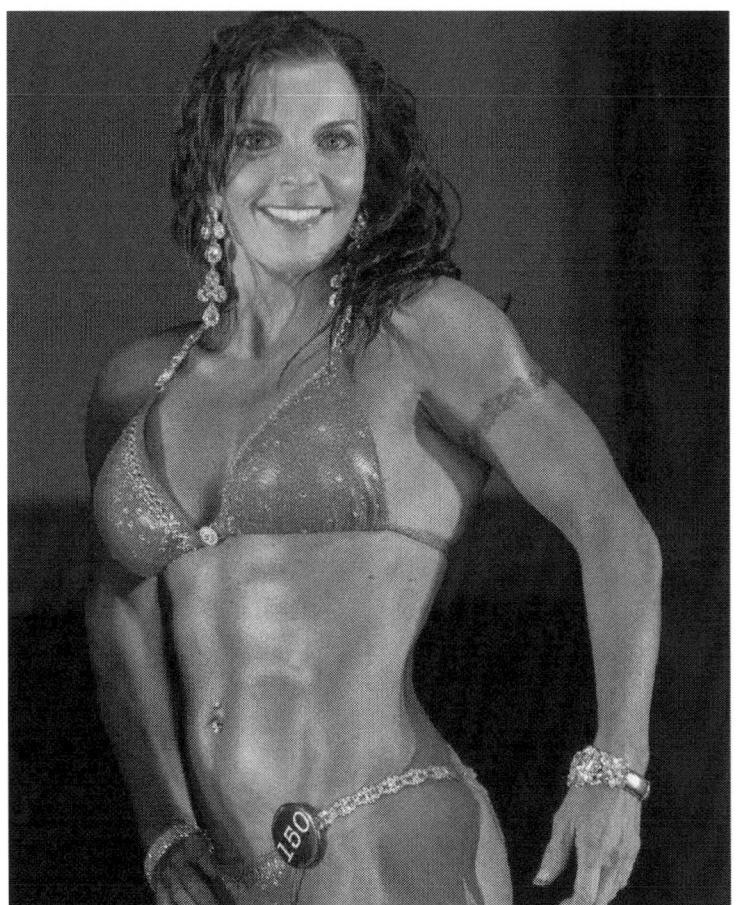

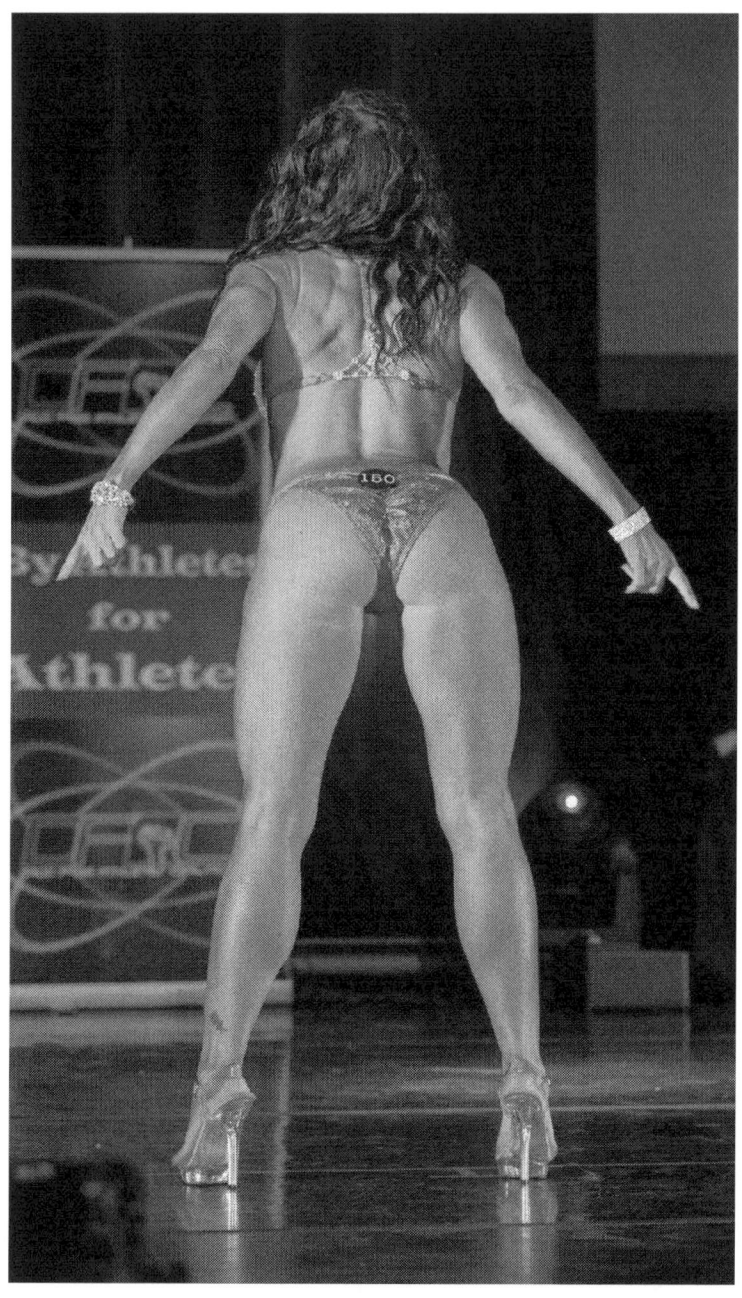

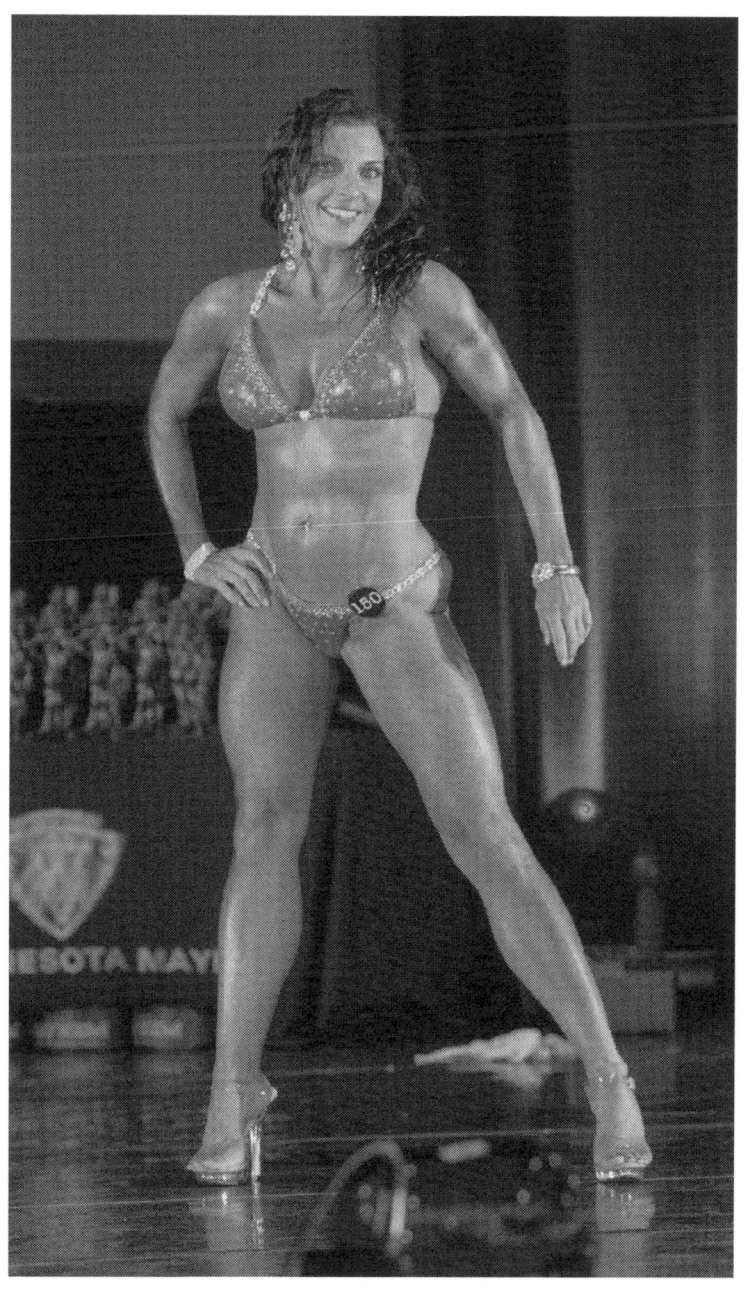

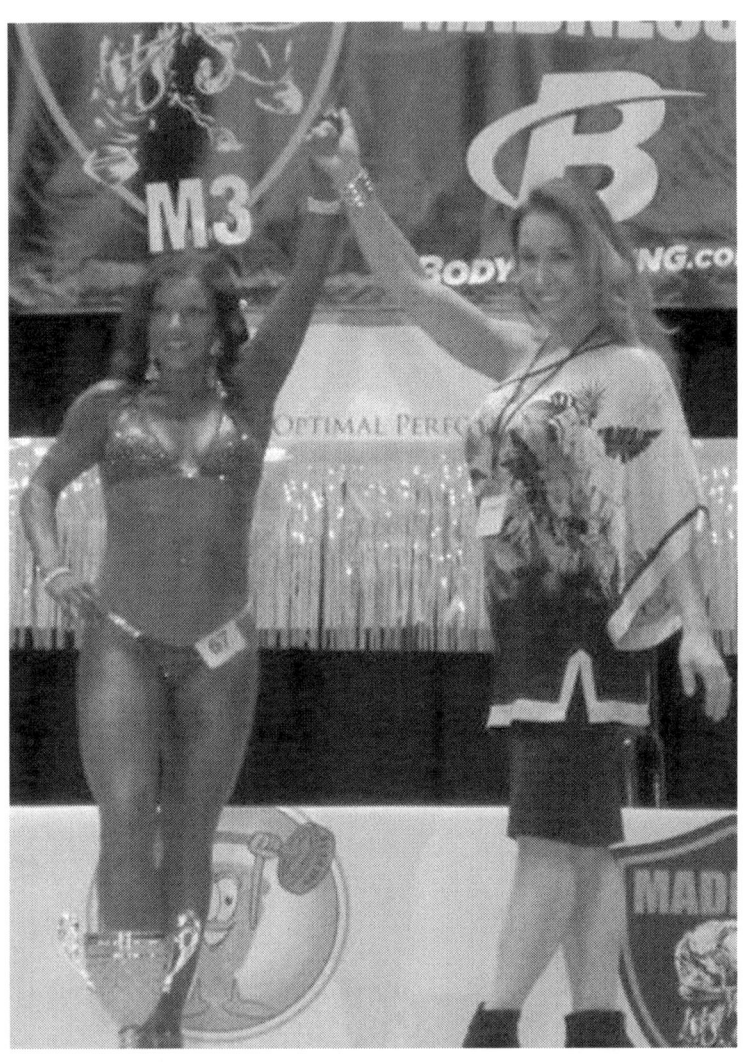

Chapter 7: TRISOmetric™ Exercises
Abdominals: Iso-Bow® Resisted Trunk Curl – Isometric and Isotonic

First, perform a trunk curl isometric exercise in three different positions which are spaced in approximately equal portions. Use an Iso-Bow® to help make the resistance easier. When you perform each isometric exercise always breathe deeply and naturally as you perform the exercise, which will be about 10 full breaths, at a rate of about 1 second per breath. Perform each exercise for no less than 7 seconds, and for no longer than 10. Try not to rest between each exercise for longer than 10 seconds. This should allow sufficient time to get into the next position. With the last isometric exercise completed, then perform a set of 10 super-slow isotonic repetitions of the trunk curl exercise. Take 10 seconds to complete the lifting phase, and 10 seconds to complete the lowering phase. Always avoid using momentum to aid the exercise.

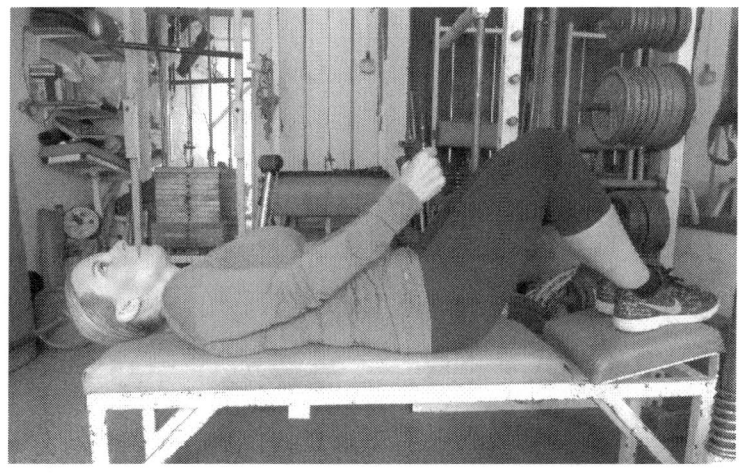

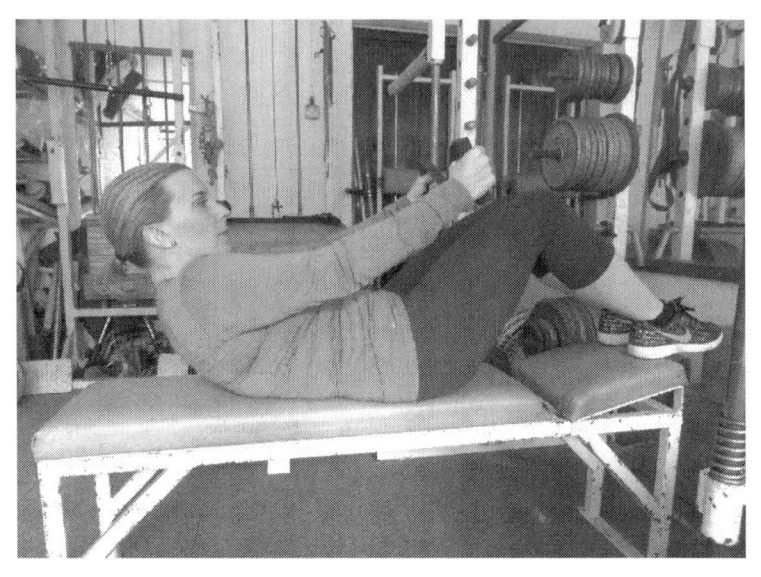

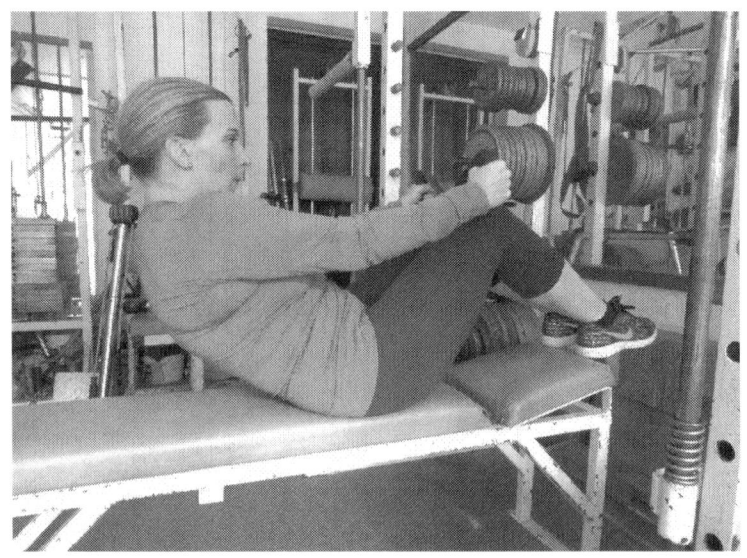

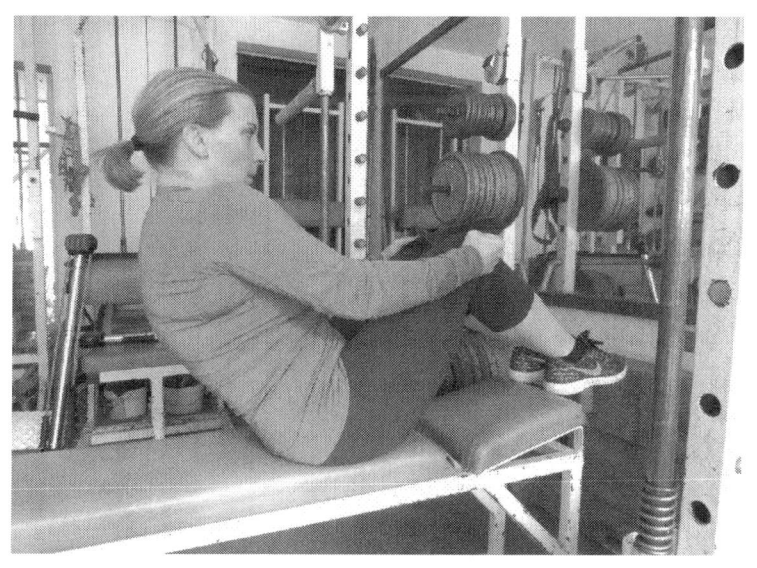

Arms - Biceps

First, perform an isometric exercise of your choice for your biceps in three different positions which are spaced in approximately equal portions. When you perform each isometric exercise always breathe deeply and naturally as you perform the exercise, which will be about 10 full breaths, at a rate of about 1 second per breath. Perform each exercise for no less than 7 seconds, and for no longer than 10. Try not to rest between each exercise for longer than 10 seconds. This should allow sufficient time to get into the next position. With the last isometric exercise completed, then perform a set of 10 super-slow isotonic repetitions of the corresponding isotonic biceps exercise. Take 10 seconds to complete the lifting phase, and 10 seconds to complete the lowering phase. Always avoid using momentum to aid the exercise.

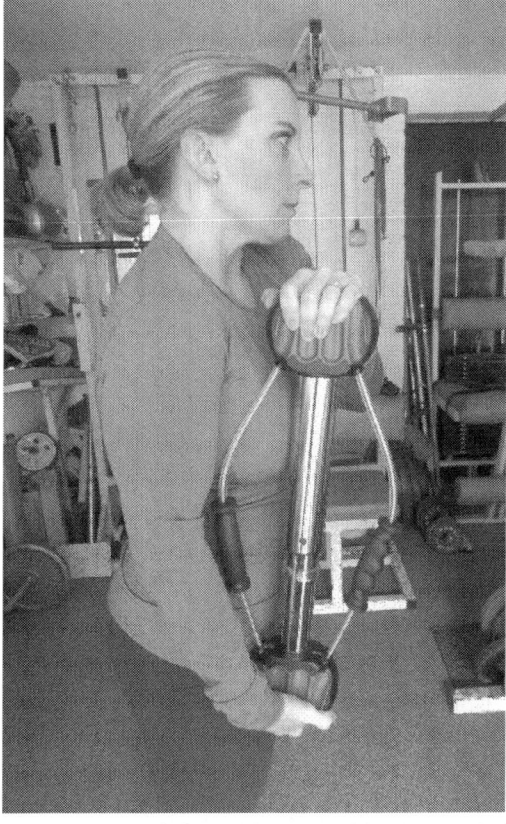

82

Isometric Biceps Exercise Example

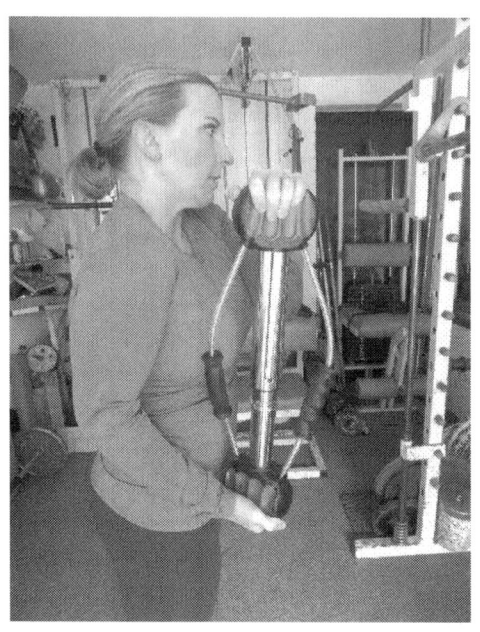

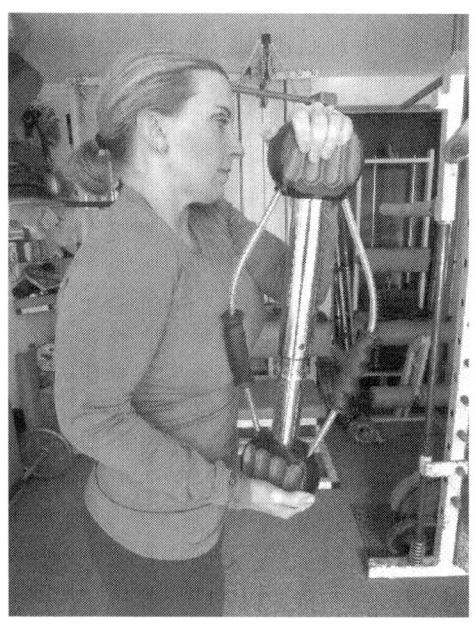

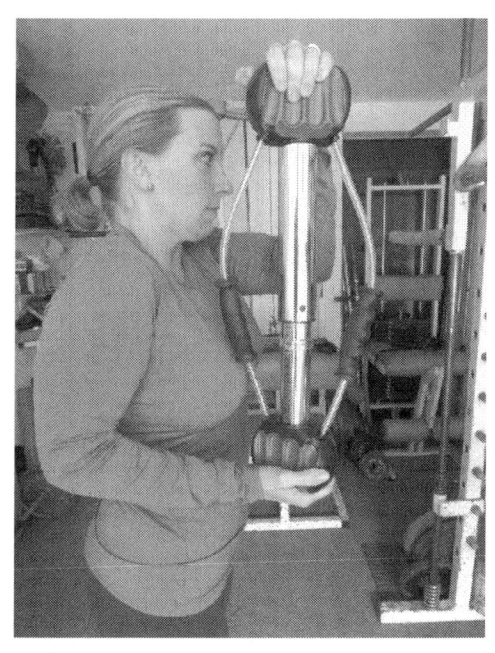

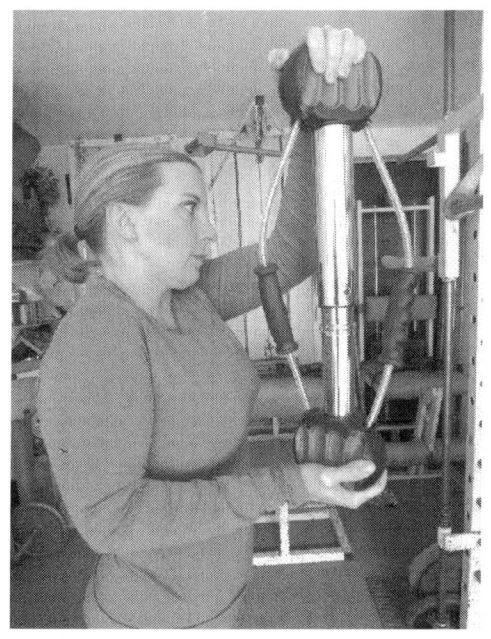

Isotonic Biceps Exercise Example

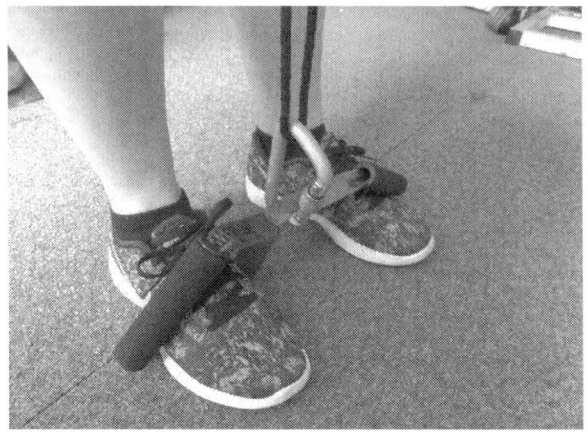

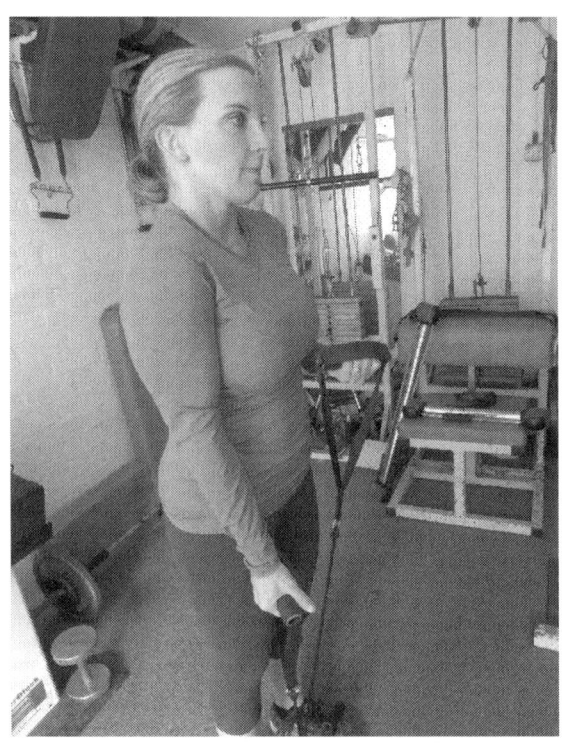

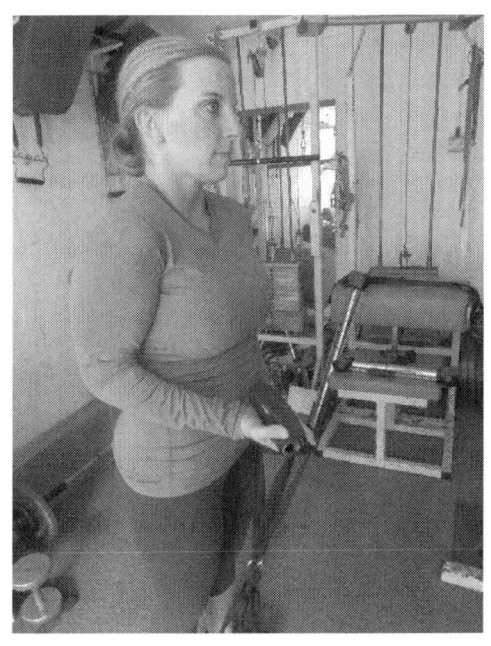

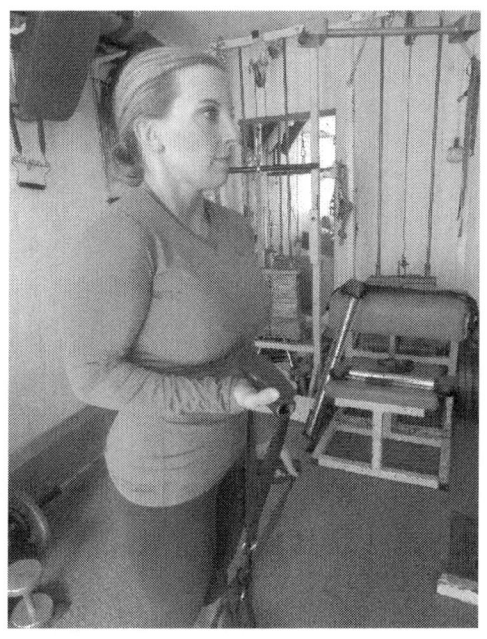

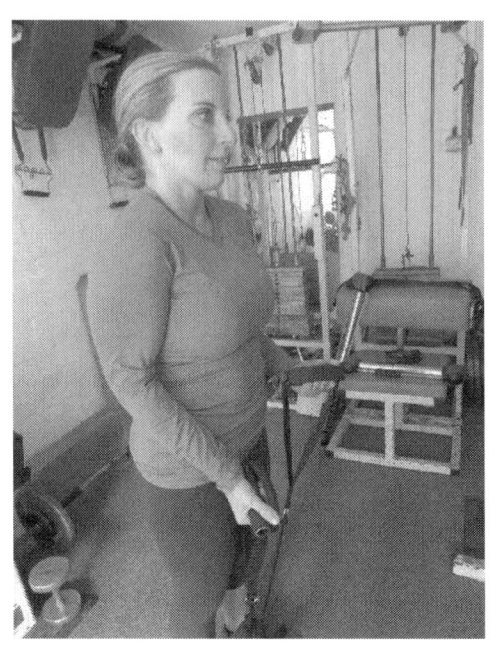

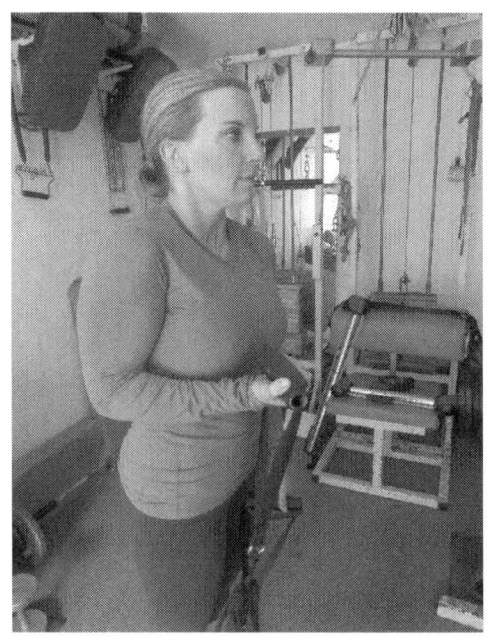

Arms - Triceps

First, perform an isometric triceps exercise of your choice in three different positions which are spaced in approximately equal portions. When you perform each isometric exercise always breathe deeply and naturally as you perform the exercise, which will be about 10 full breaths, at a rate of about 1 second per breath. Perform each exercise for no less than 7 seconds, and for no longer than 10. Try not to rest between each exercise for longer than 10 seconds. This should allow sufficient time to get into the next position. With the last isometric exercise completed, then perform a set of 10 super-slow isotonic repetitions of the corresponding isotonic triceps exercise. Take 10 seconds to complete the lifting phase, and 10 seconds to complete the lowering phase. Always avoid using momentum to aid the exercise.

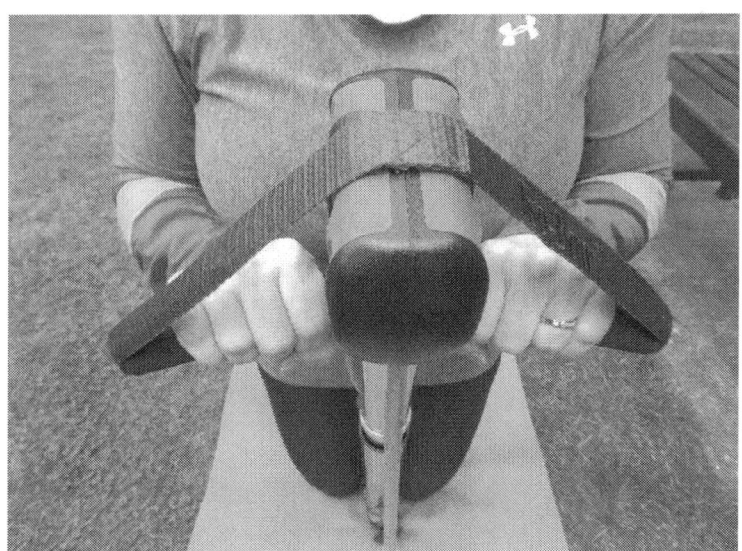

Isometric Triceps Exercise Example

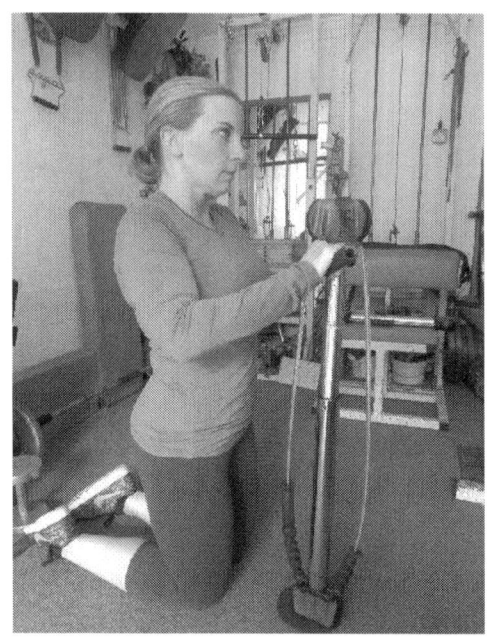

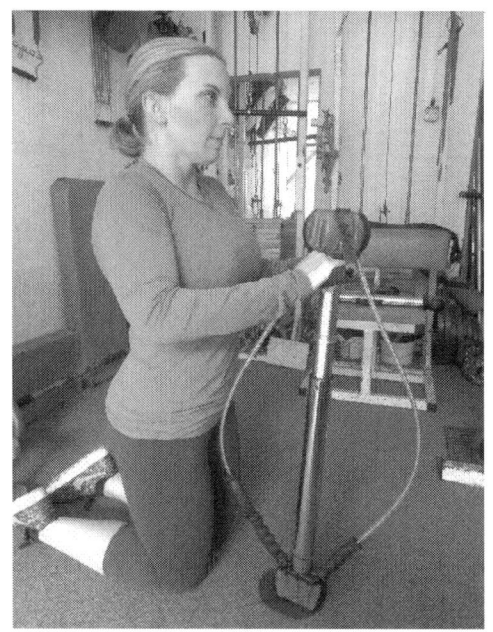

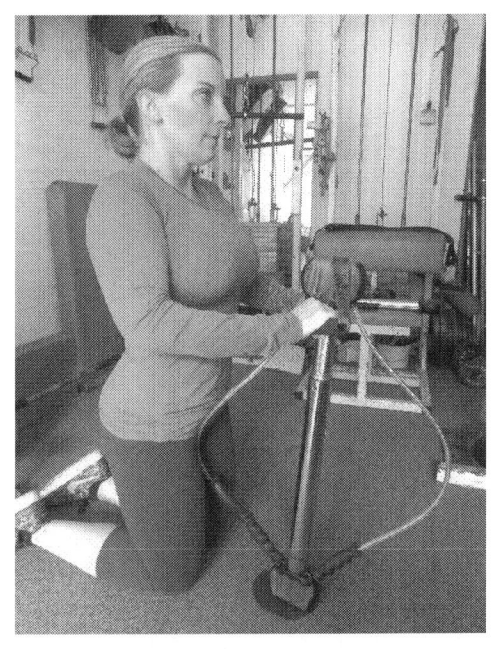

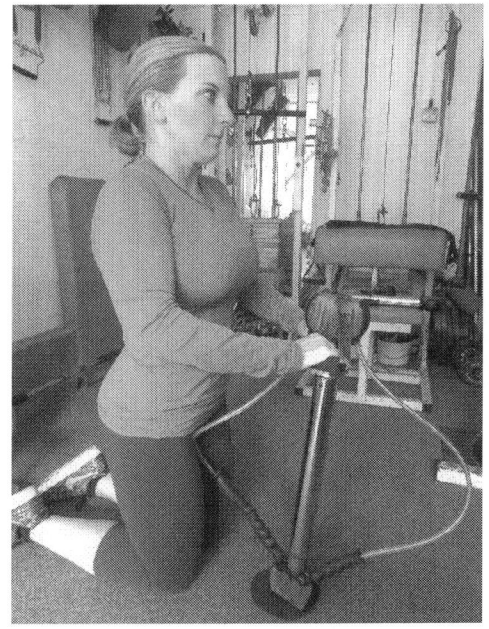

Isotonic Triceps Exercise Example

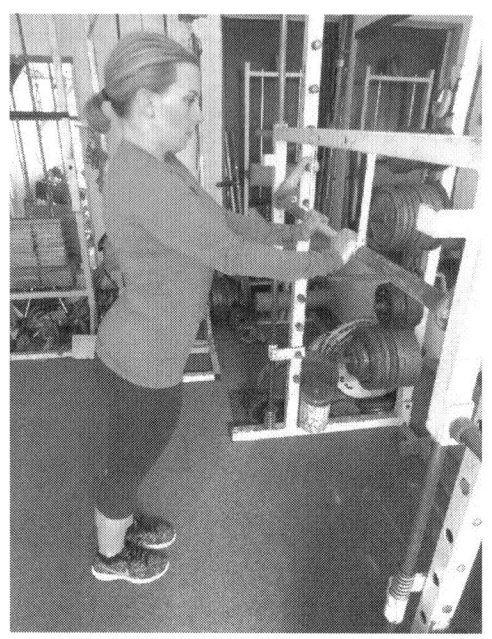

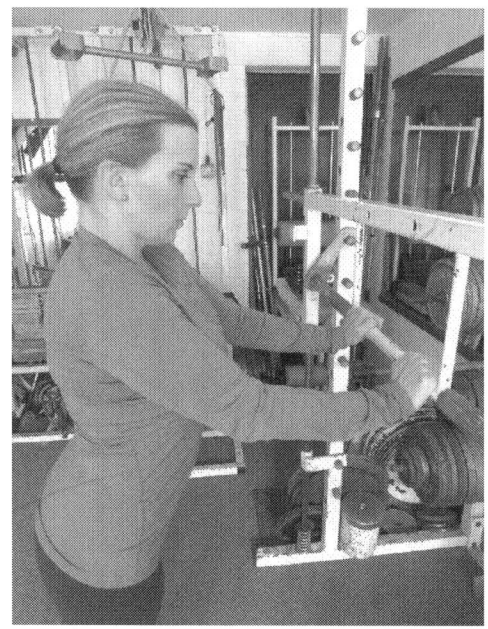

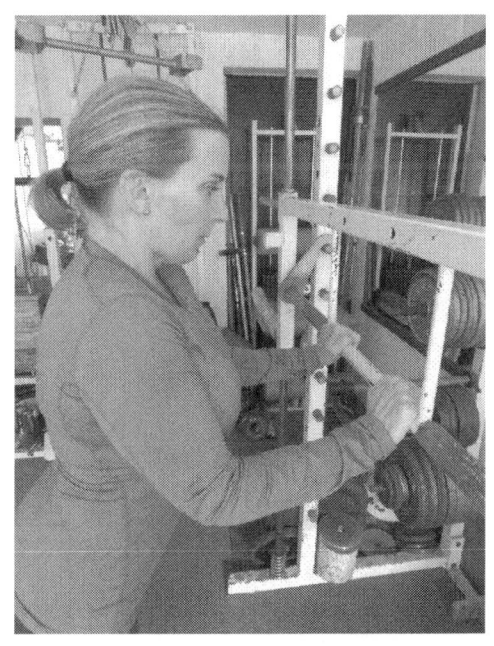

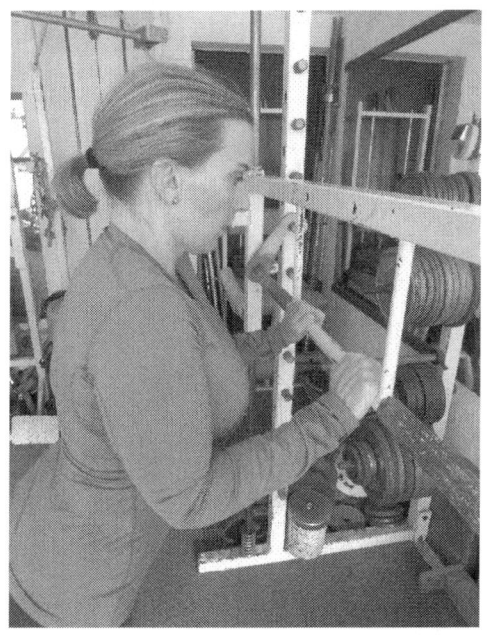

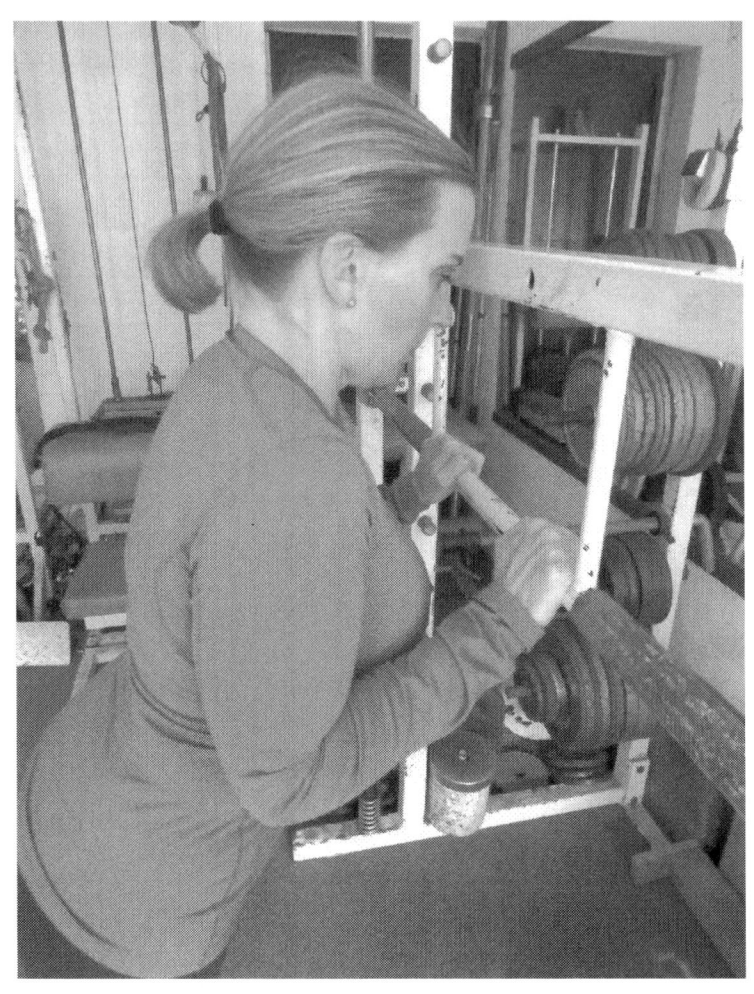

Back - Lower

First, perform an isometric lower back exercise of your choice in three different positions which are spaced in approximately equal portions. When you perform each isometric exercise always breathe deeply and naturally as you perform the exercise, which will be about 10 full breaths, at a rate of about 1 second per breath. Perform each exercise for no less than 7 seconds, and for no longer than 10. Try not to rest between each exercise for longer than 10 seconds. This should allow sufficient time to get into the next position. With the last isometric exercise completed, then perform a set of 10 super-slow isotonic repetitions of the corresponding isotonic lower back exercise. Take 10 seconds to complete the lifting phase, and 10 seconds to complete the lowering phase. Always avoid using momentum to aid the exercise.

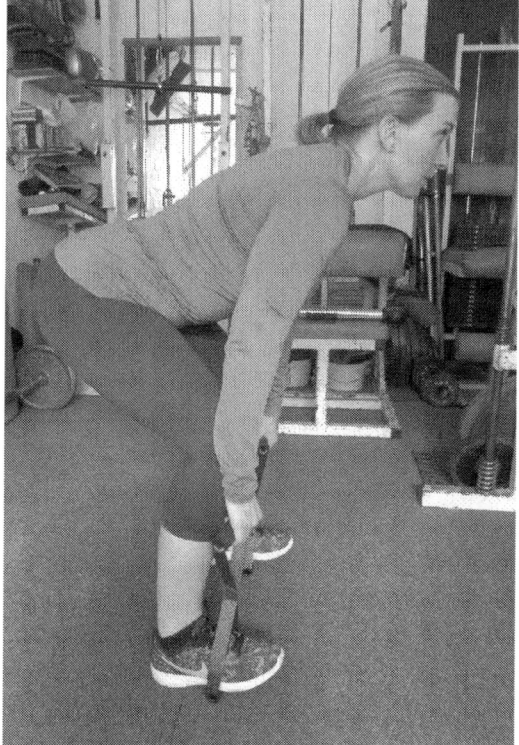

Isometric Lower Back Exercise Example

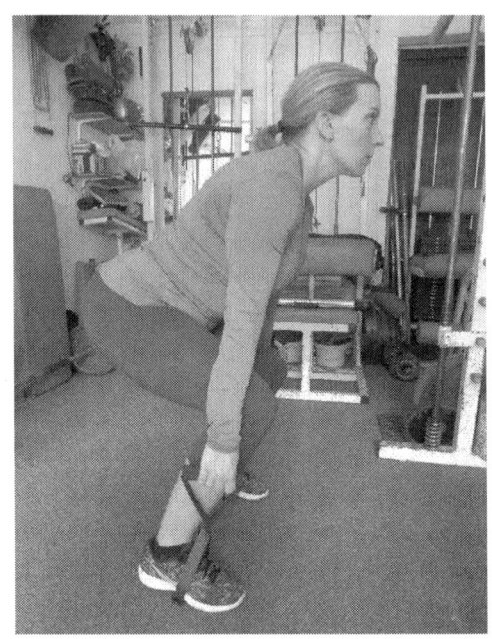

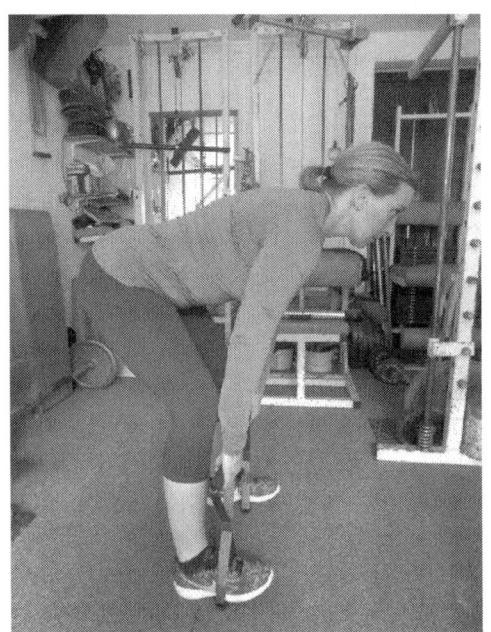

Isotonic Lower Back Exercise Example A

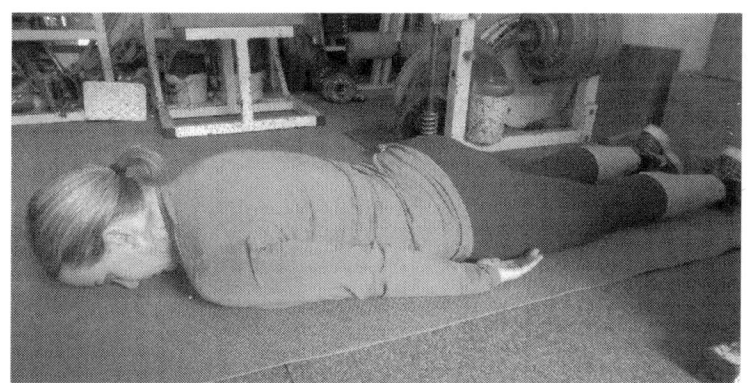

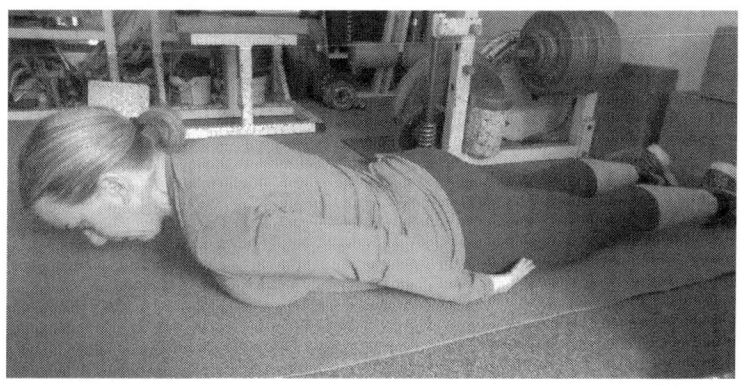

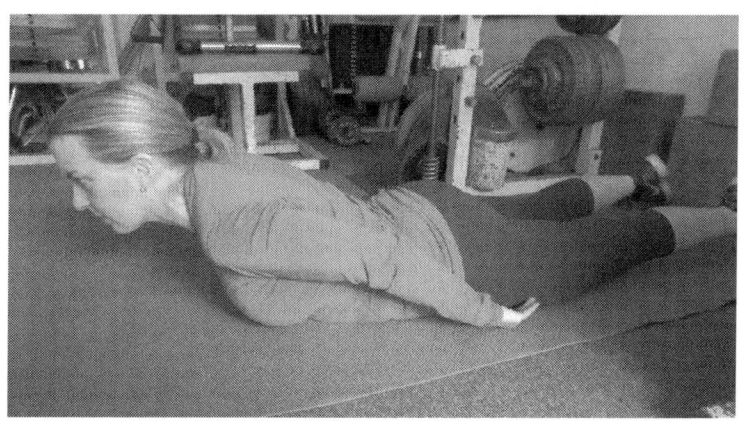

Isotonic Lower Back Exercise Example B

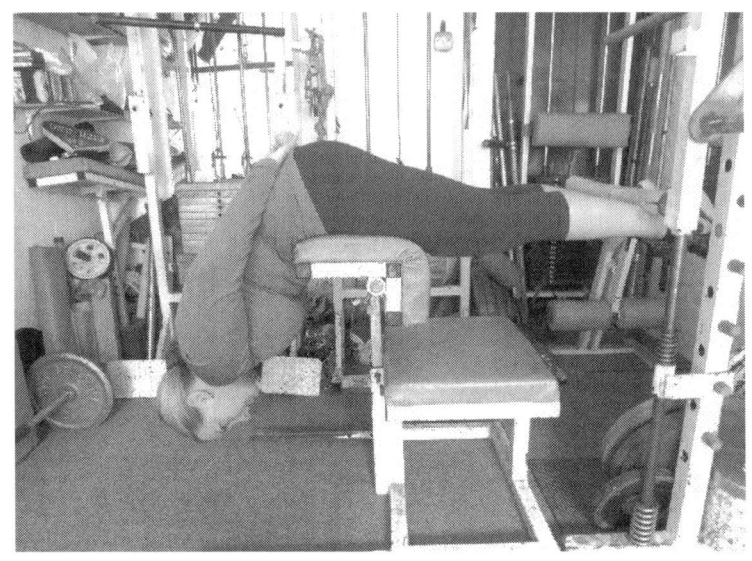

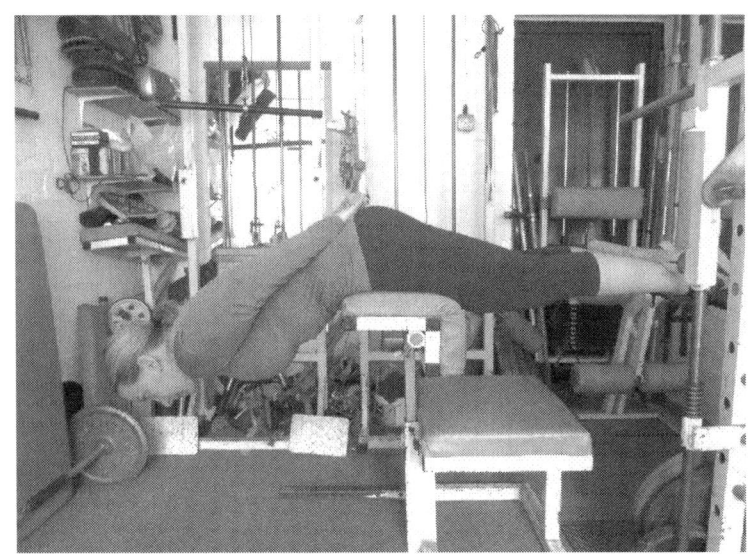

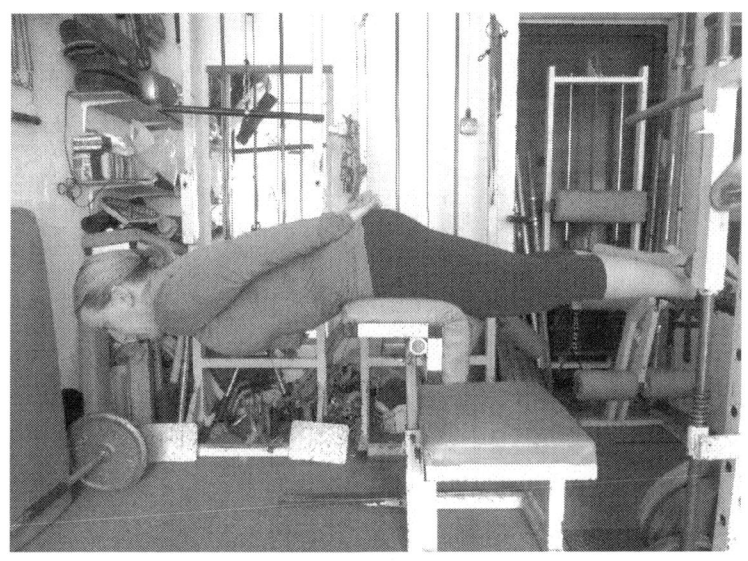

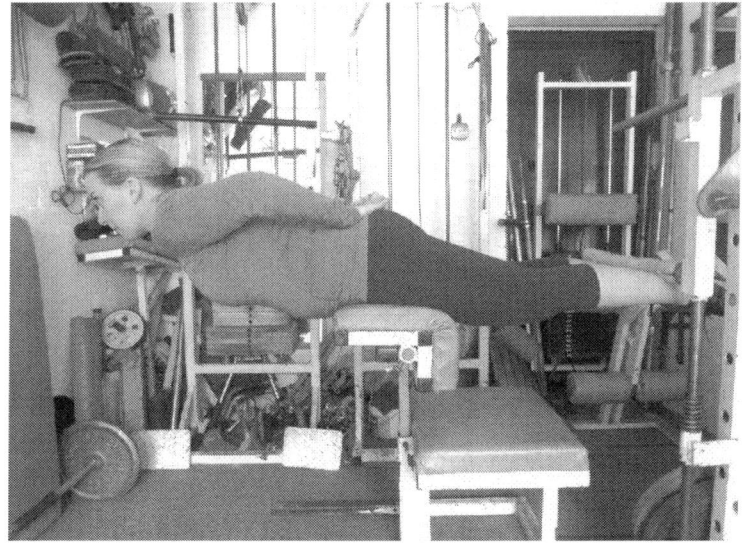

Back - Upper

First, perform an isometric upper back exercise of your choice in three different positions which are spaced in approximately equal portions. When you perform each isometric exercise always breathe deeply and naturally as you perform the exercise, which will be about 10 full breaths, at a rate of about 1 second per breath. Perform each exercise for no less than 7 seconds, and for no longer than 10. Try not to rest between each exercise for longer than 10 seconds. This should allow sufficient time to get into the next position. With the last isometric exercise completed, then perform a set of 10 super-slow isotonic repetitions of the corresponding isotonic upper back exercise. Take 10 seconds to complete the lifting phase, and 10 seconds to complete the lowering phase. Always avoid using momentum to aid the exercise.

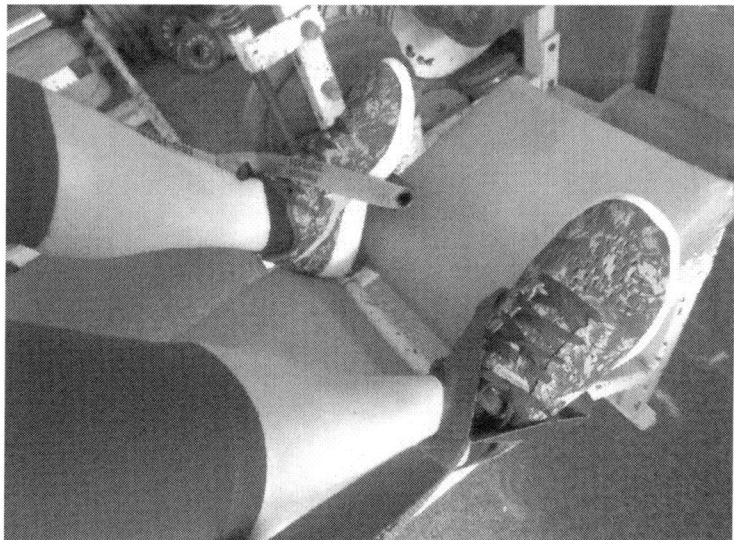

Isometric Upper Back Exercise Example

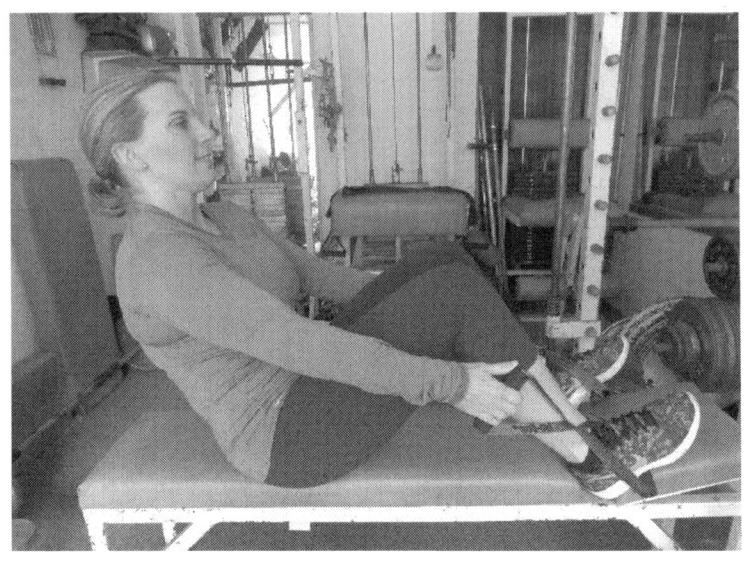

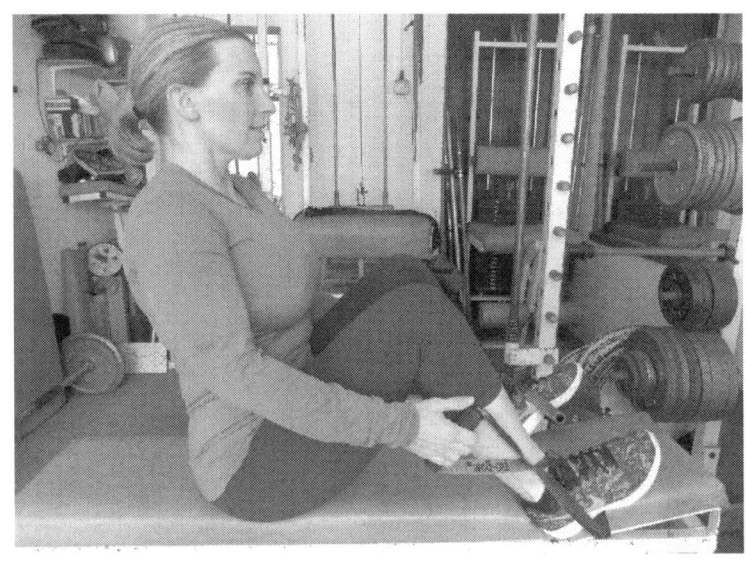

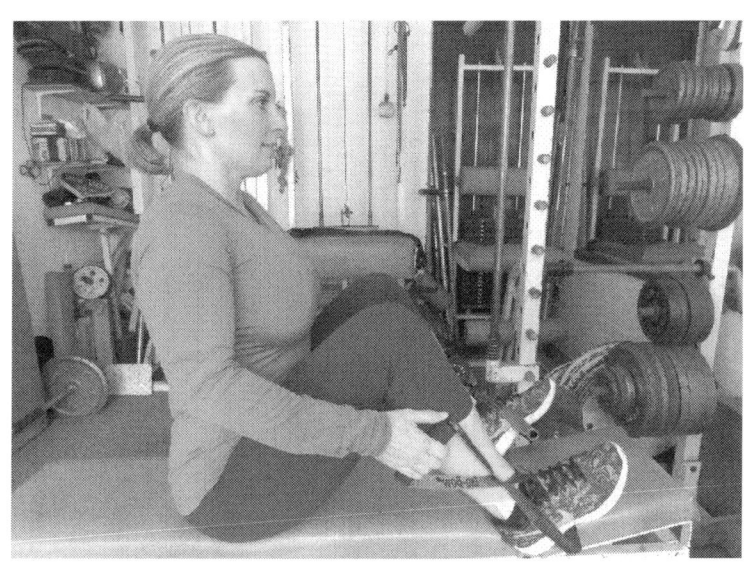

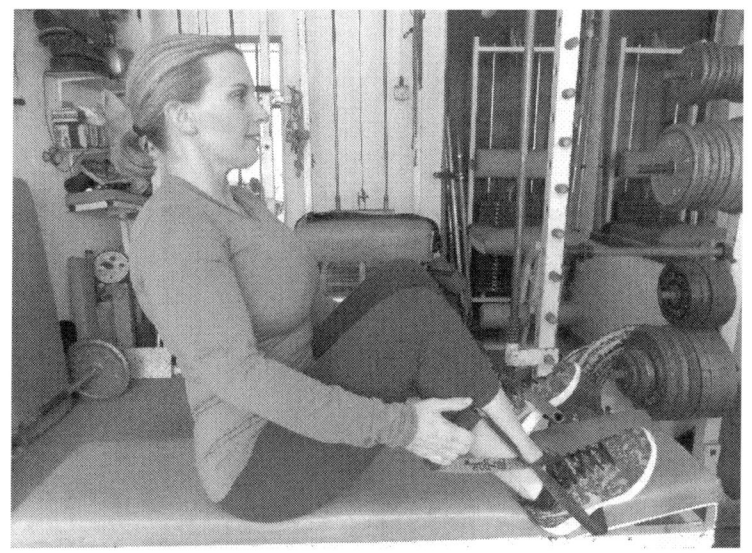

Isotonic Upper Back Exercise Example

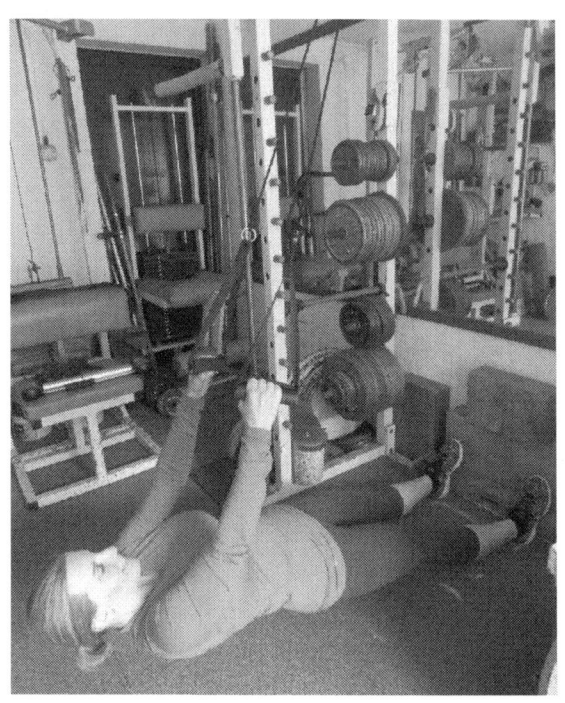

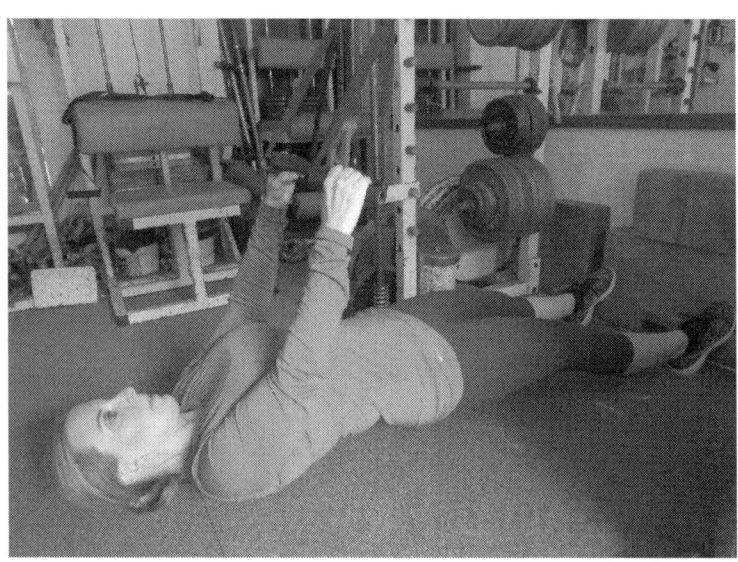

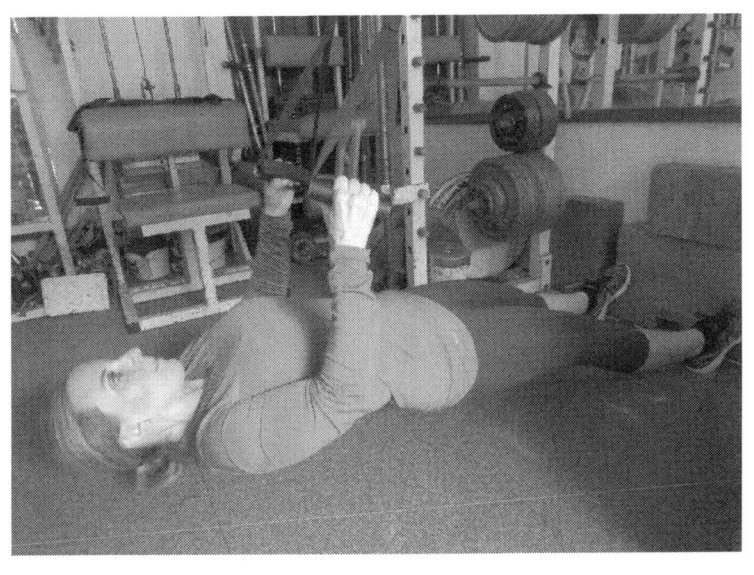

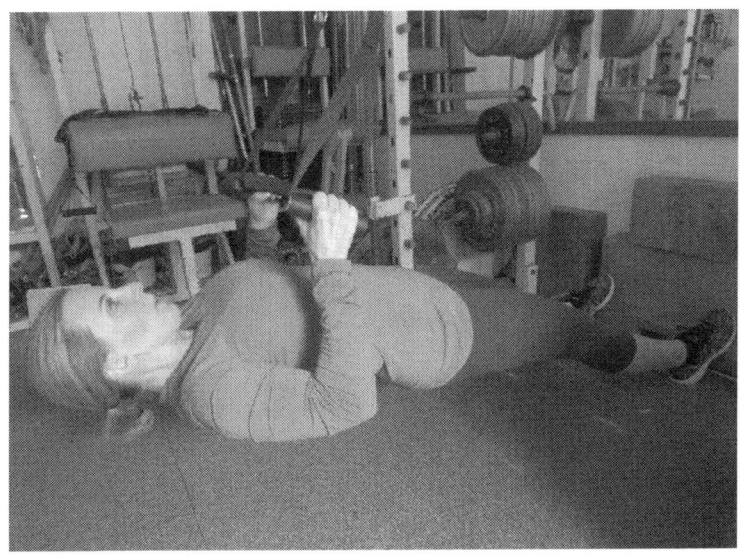

Chest

First, perform an isometric chest exercise of your choice in three different positions which are spaced in approximately equal portions. When you perform each isometric exercise always breathe deeply and naturally as you perform the exercise, which will be about 10 full breaths, at a rate of about 1 second per breath. Perform each exercise for no less than 7 seconds, and for no longer than 10. Try not to rest between each exercise for longer than 10 seconds. This should allow sufficient time to get into the next position. With the last isometric exercise completed, then perform a set of 10 super-slow isotonic repetitions of the corresponding isotonic chest exercise. Take 10 seconds to complete the lifting phase, and 10 seconds to complete the lowering phase. Always avoid using momentum to aid the exercise.

Isometric Chest Exercise Example A

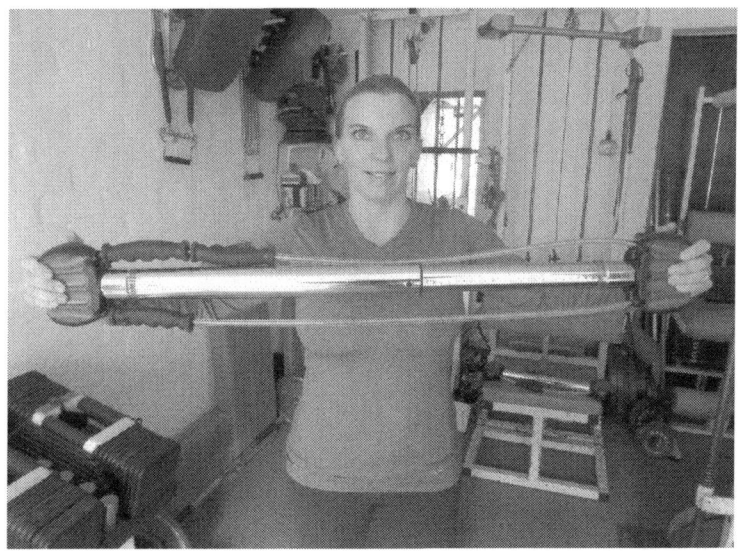

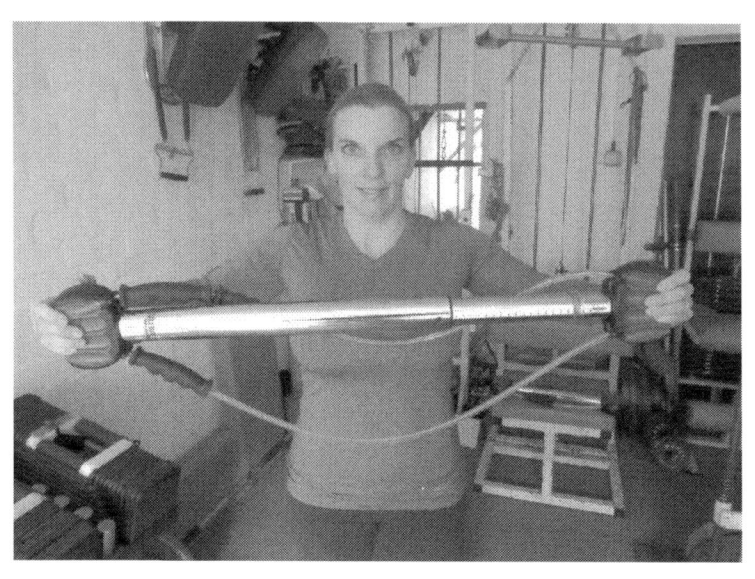

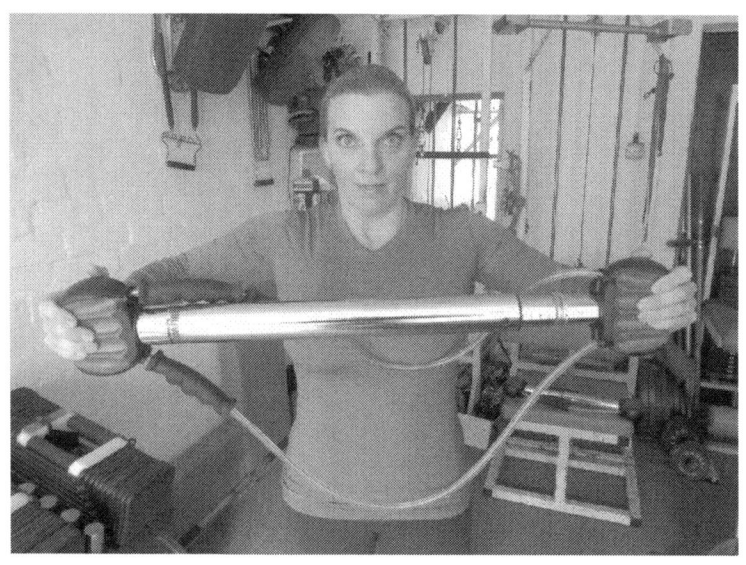

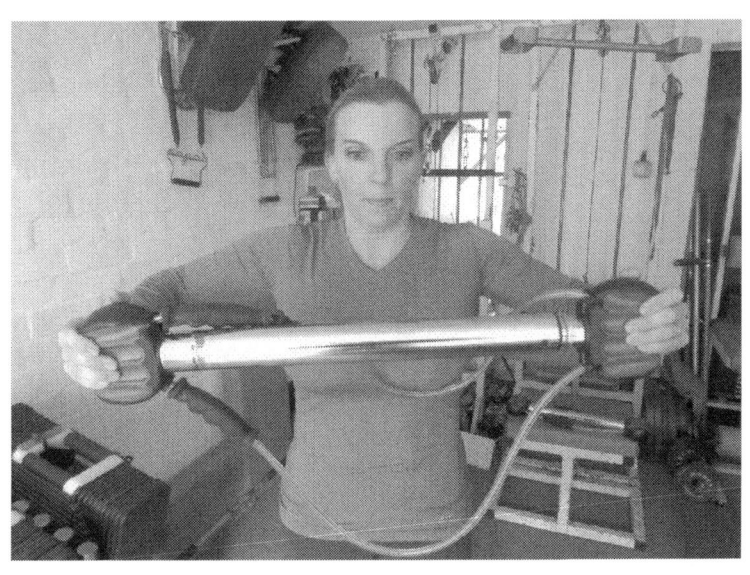

Isometric Chest Exercise Example B

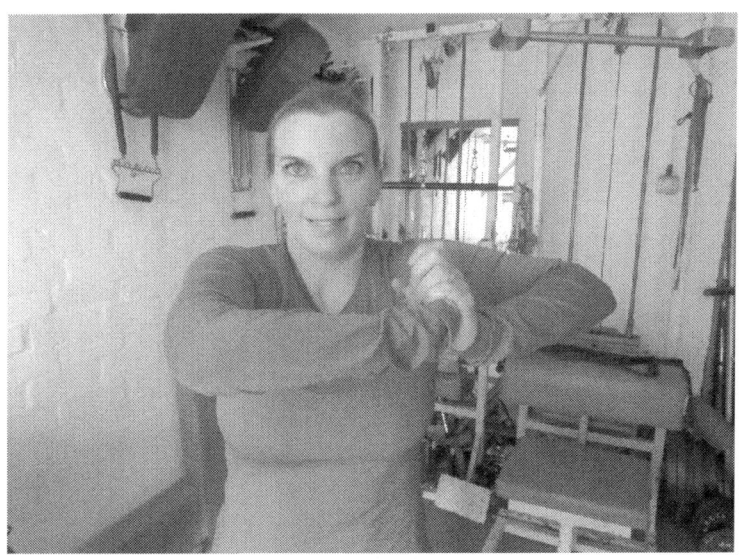

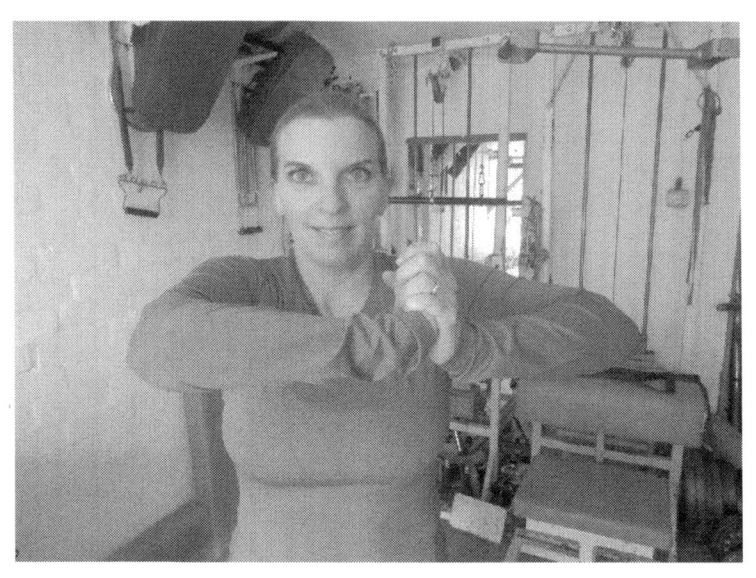

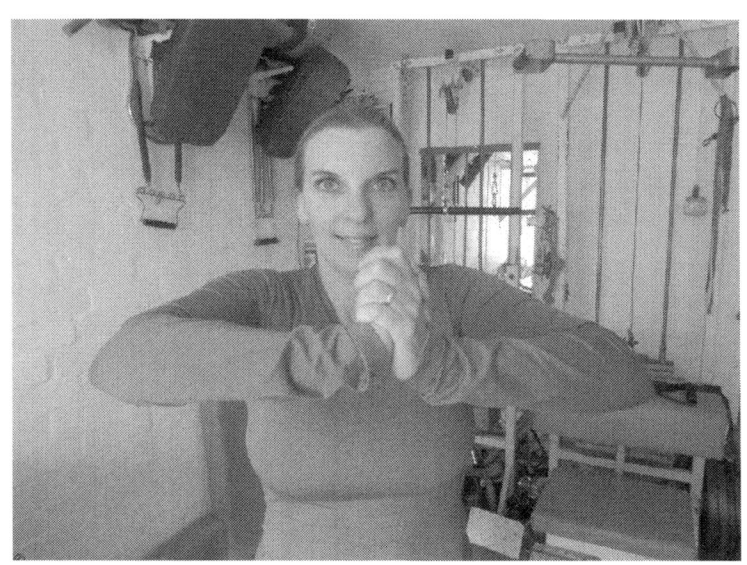

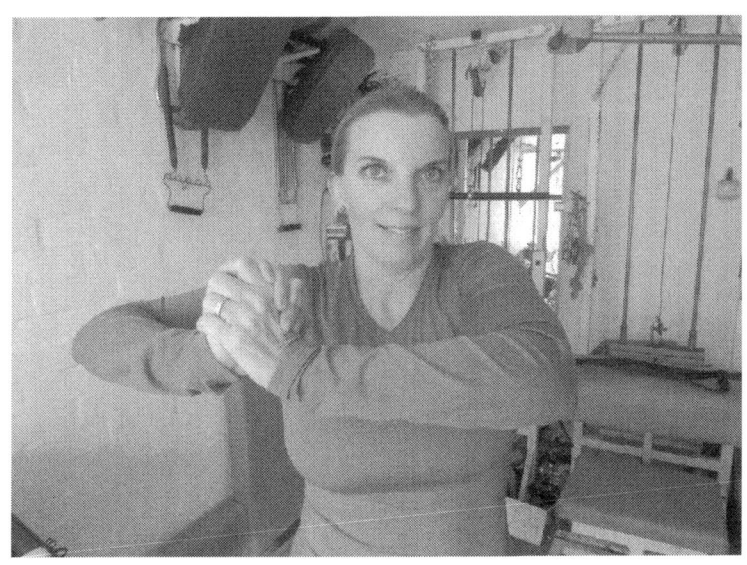

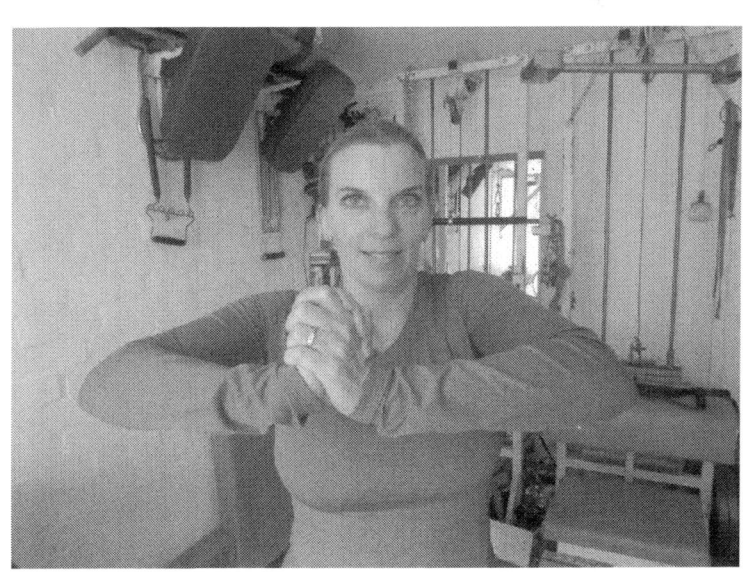

Isotonic Chest Exercise Example A

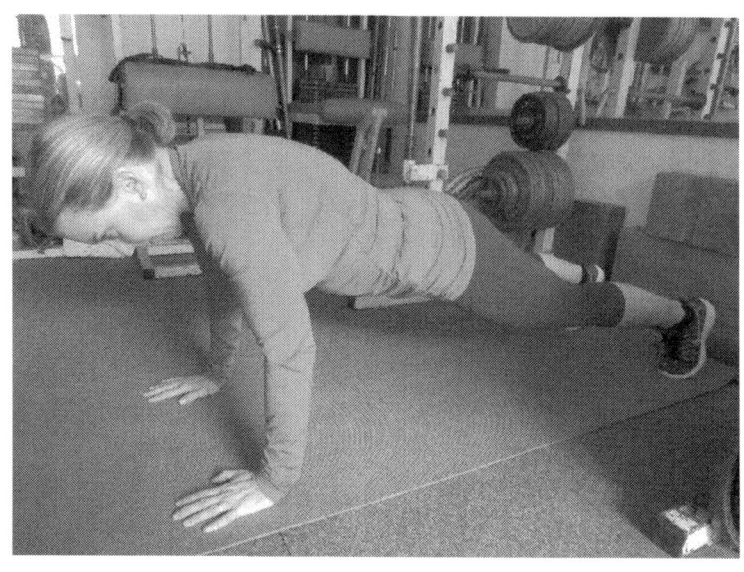

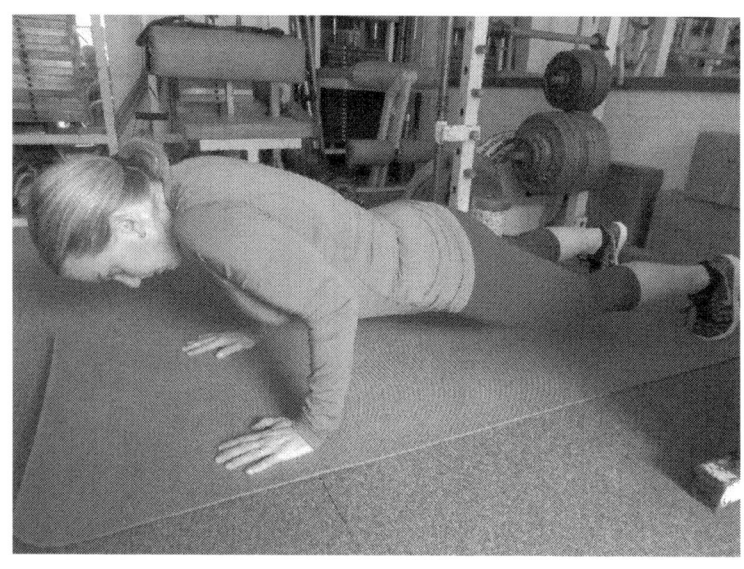

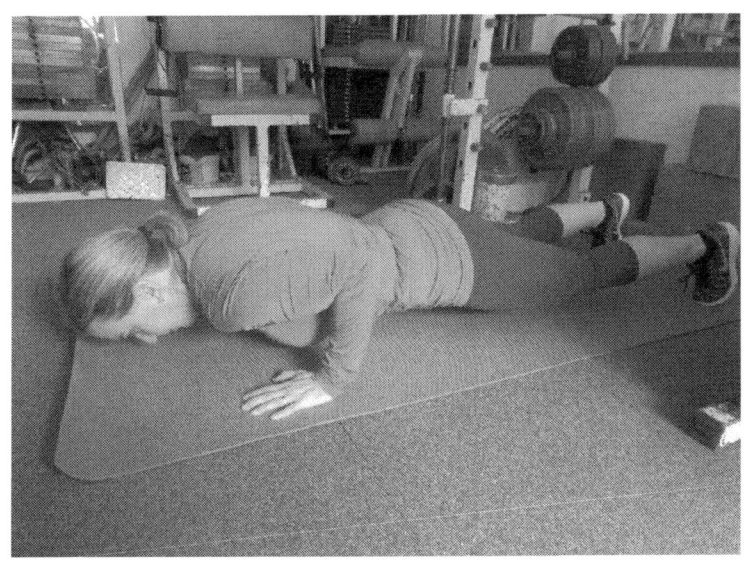

Isotonic Chest Exercise Example B

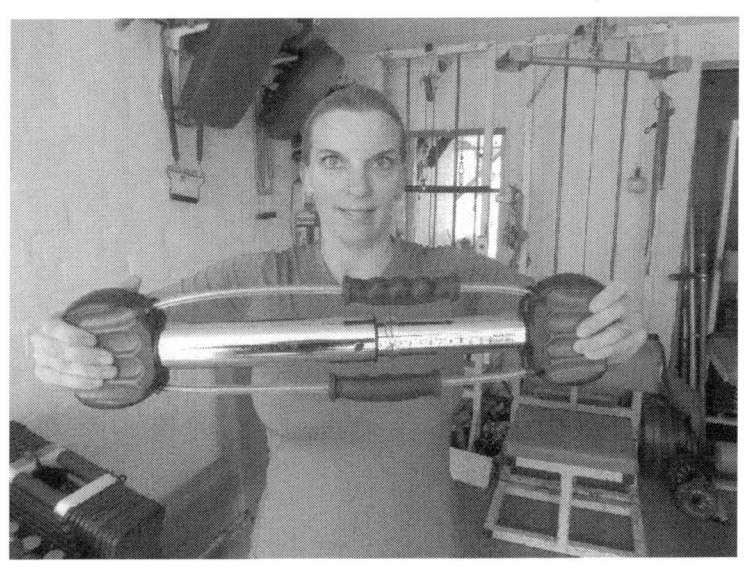

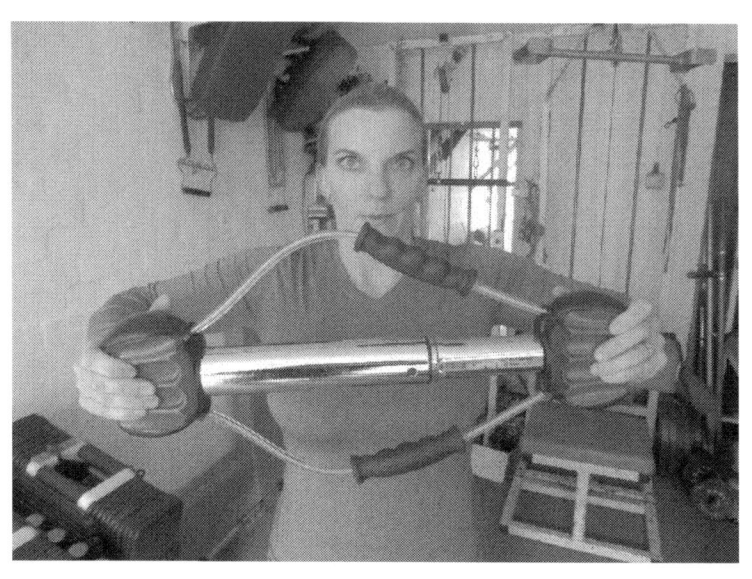

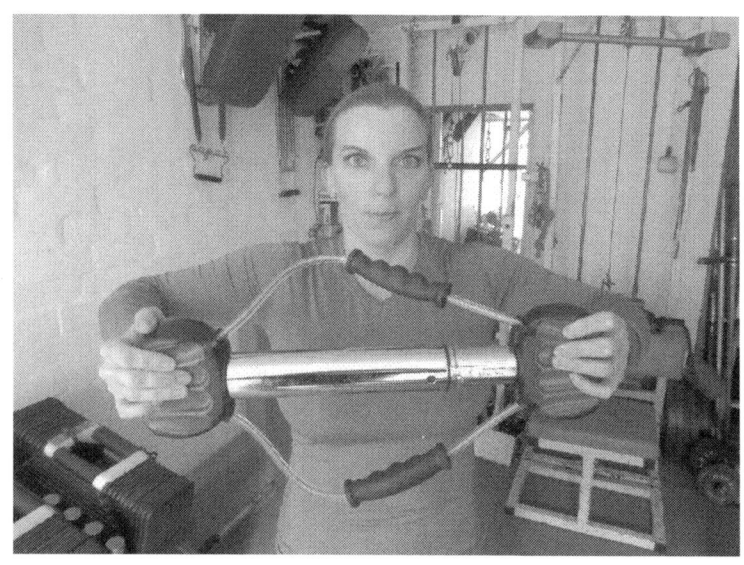

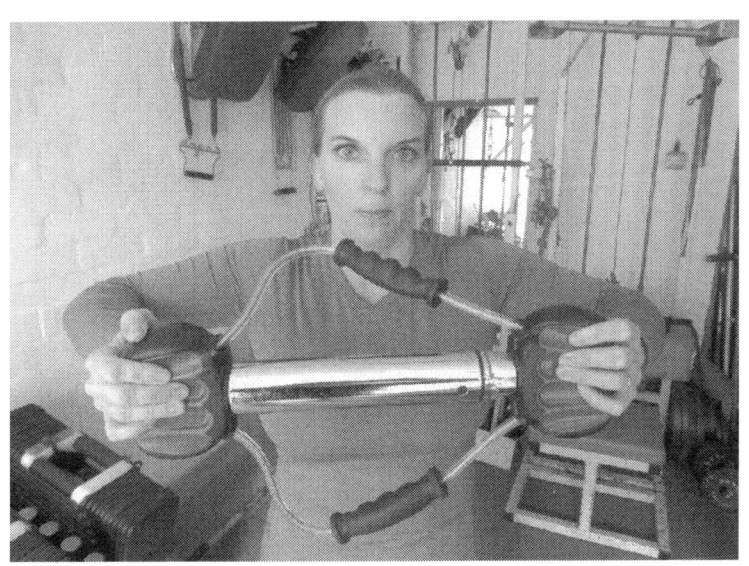

Legs - Thighs

First, perform an isometric thigh exercise of your choice in three different positions which are spaced in approximately equal portions. When you perform each isometric exercise always breathe deeply and naturally as you perform the exercise, which will be about 10 full breaths, at a rate of about 1 second per breath. Perform each exercise for no less than 7 seconds, and for no longer than 10. Try not to rest between each exercise for longer than 10 seconds. This should allow sufficient time to get into the next position. With the last isometric exercise completed, then perform a set of 10 super-slow isotonic repetitions of the corresponding isotonic thigh exercise. Take 10 seconds to complete the lifting phase, and 10 seconds to complete the lowering phase. Always avoid using momentum to aid the exercise.

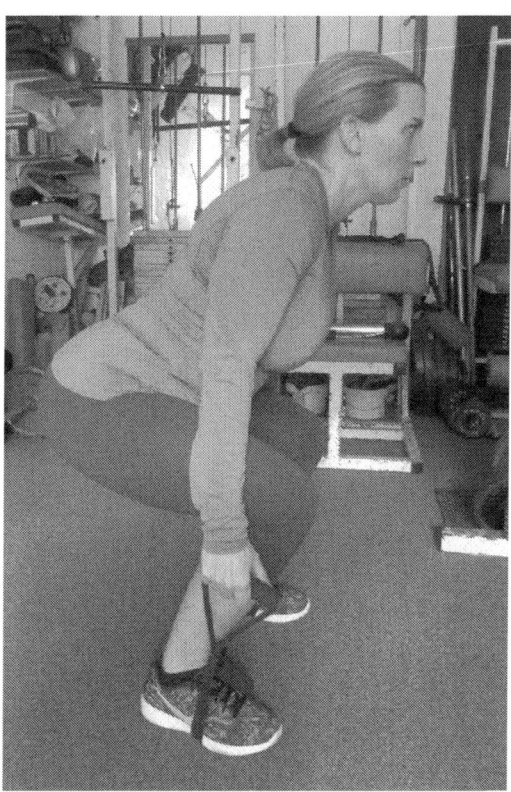

Isometric Thigh Exercise Example

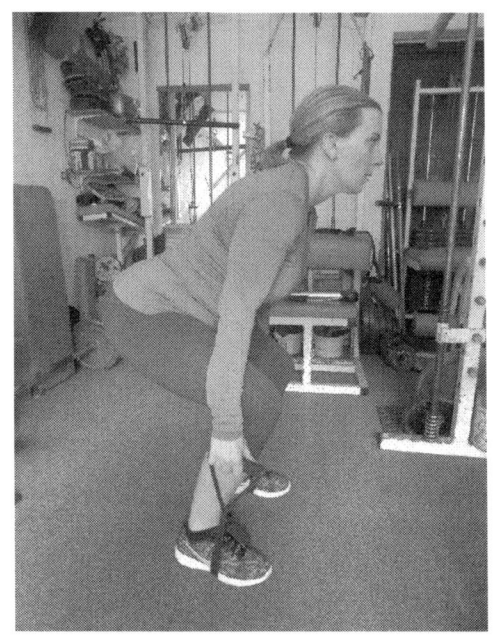

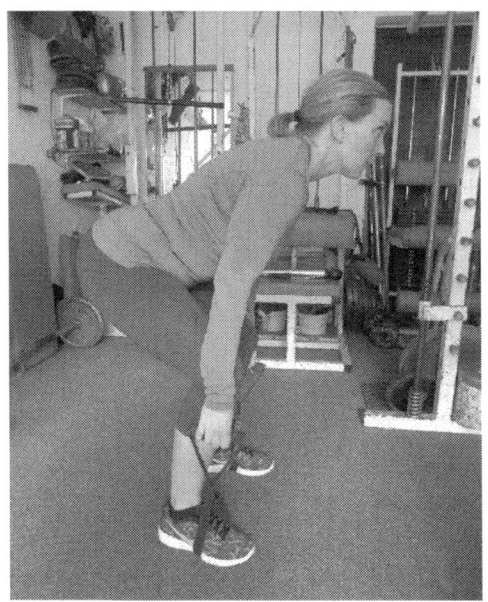

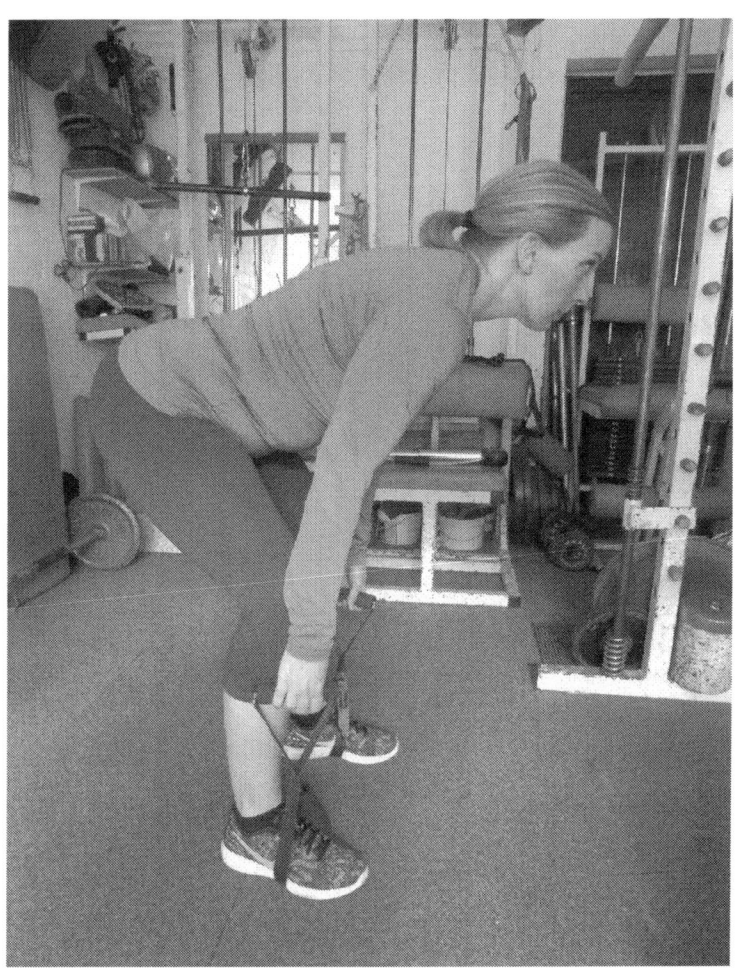

Isotonic Thigh Exercise Example

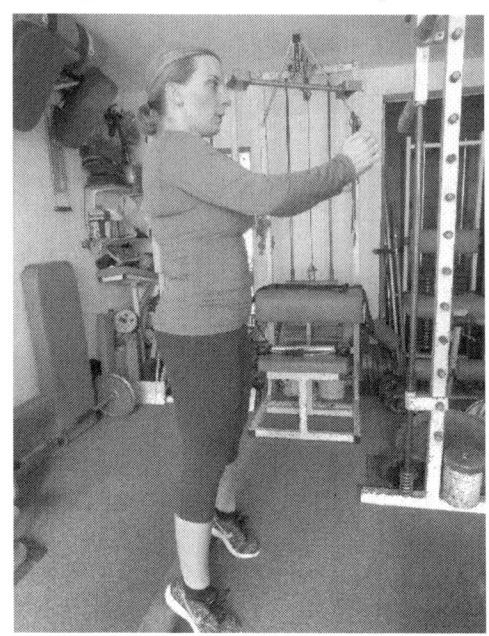

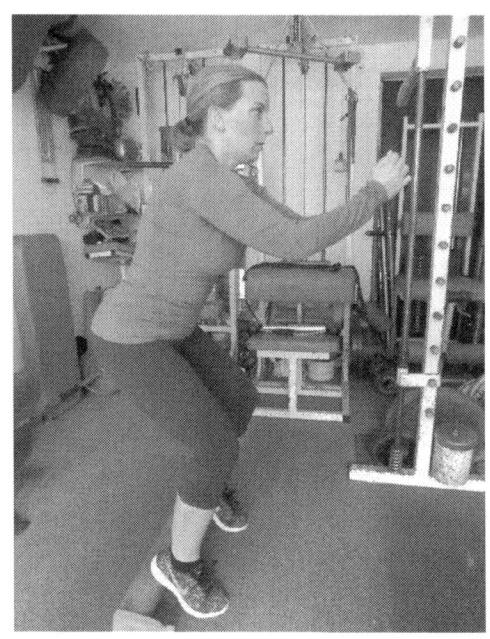

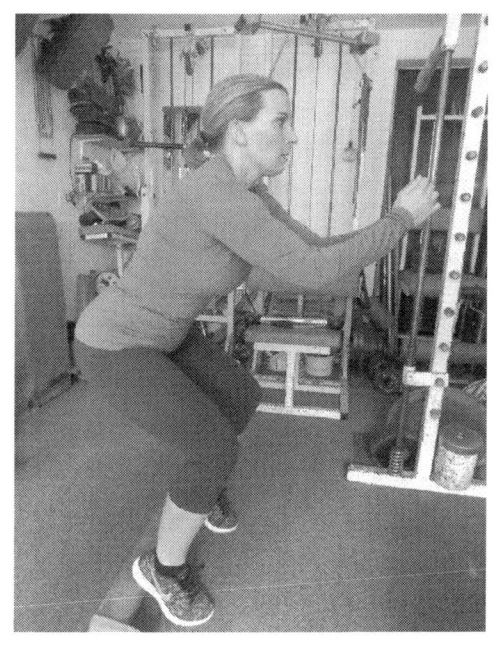

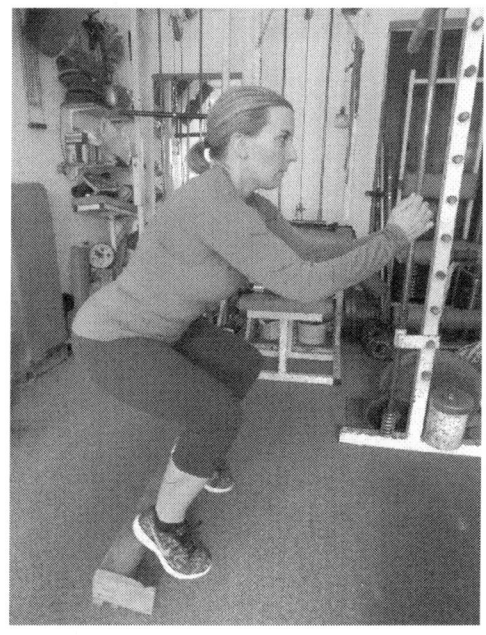

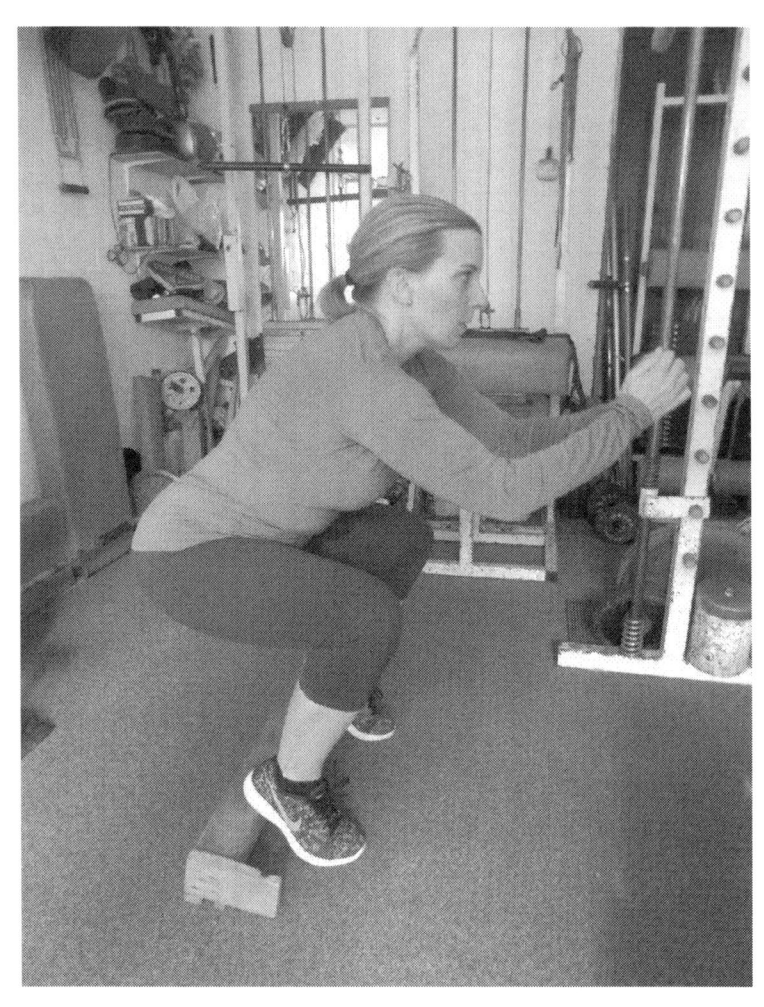

Legs - Calf's

First, perform an isometric *calf* exercise of your choice in three different positions which are spaced in approximately equal portions. When you perform each isometric exercise always breathe deeply and naturally as you perform the exercise, which will be about 10 full breaths, at a rate of about 1 second per breath. Perform each exercise for no less than 7 seconds, and for no longer than 10. Try not to rest between each exercise for longer than 10 seconds. This should allow sufficient time to get into the next position. With the last isometric exercise completed, then perform a set of 10 super-slow isotonic repetitions of the corresponding isotonic calf exercise. Take 10 seconds to complete the lifting phase, and 10 seconds to complete the lowering phase. Always avoid using momentum to aid the exercise.

Isometric Calf Exercise Example

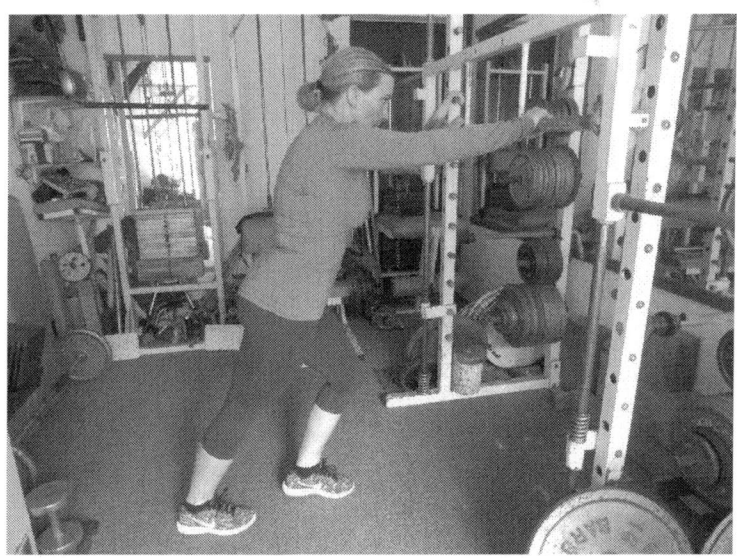

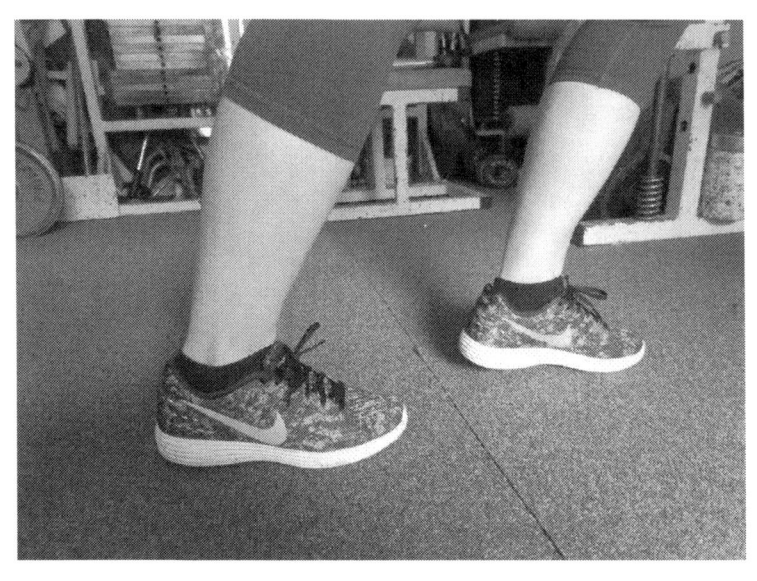

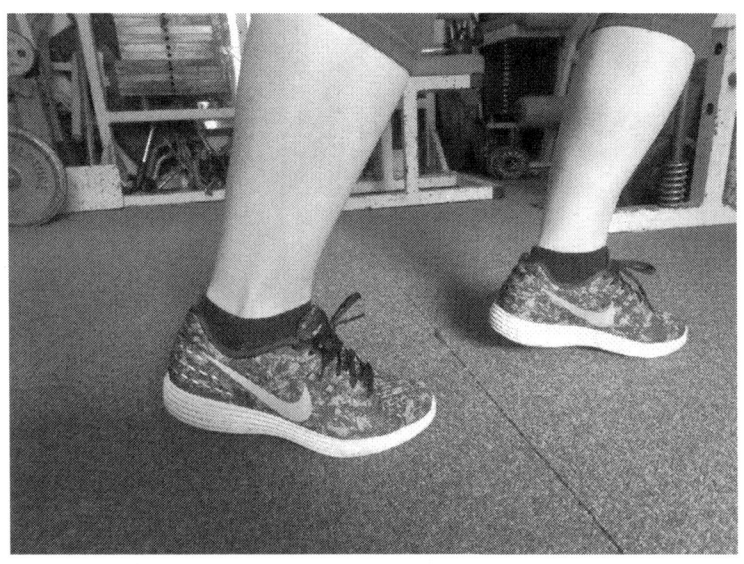

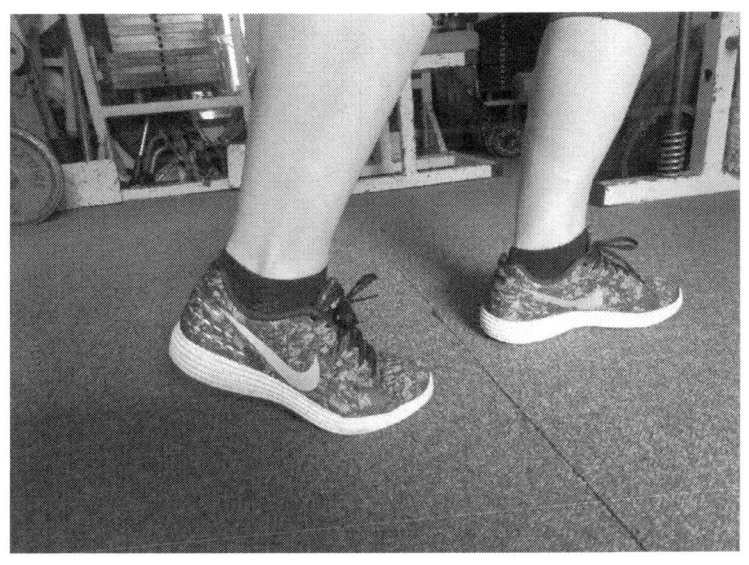

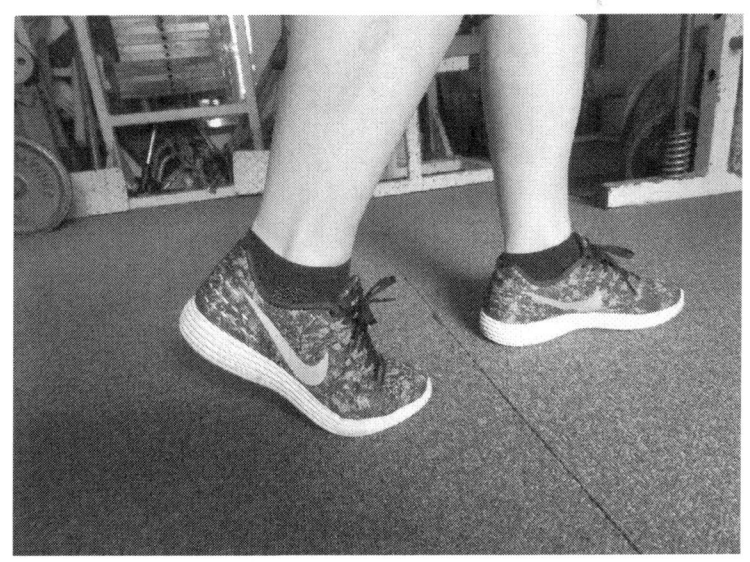

Isotonic Calf Exercise Example

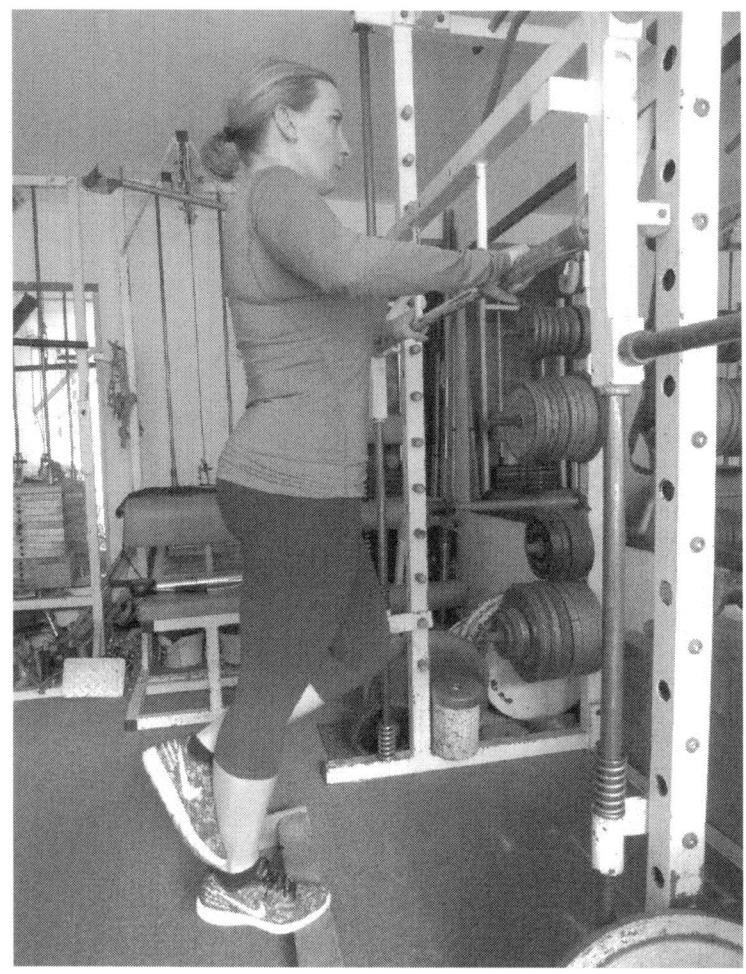

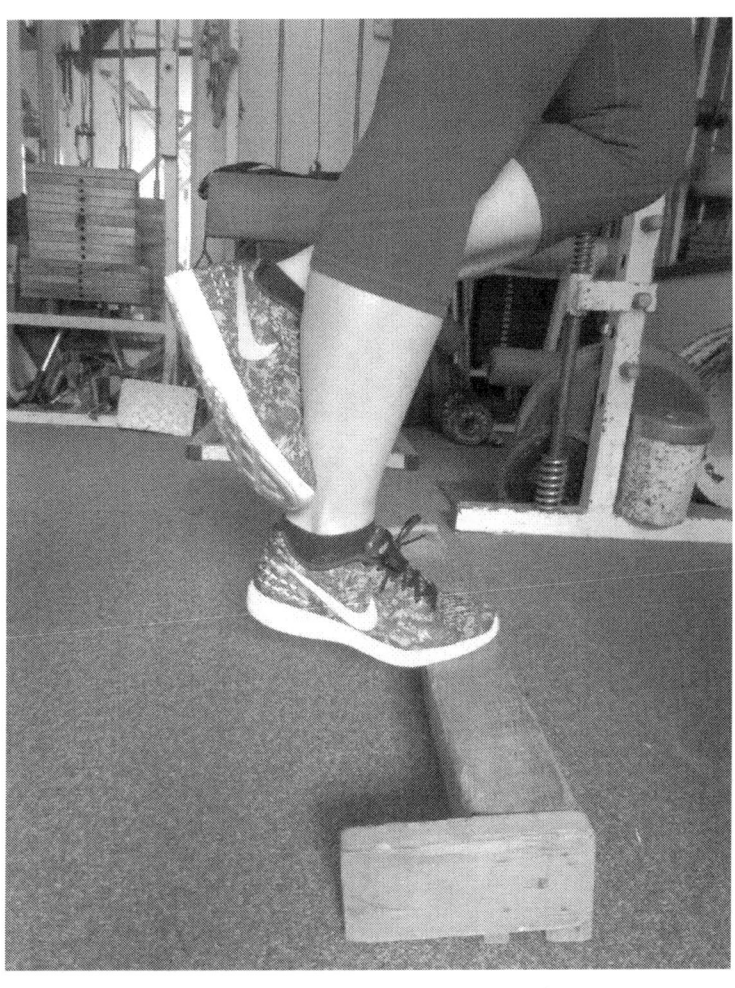

Shoulders

First, perform an isometric *shoulder* exercise of your choice in three different positions which are spaced in approximately equal portions. When you perform each isometric exercise always breathe deeply and naturally as you perform the exercise, which will be about 10 full breaths, at a rate of about 1 second per breath. Perform each exercise for no less than 7 seconds, and for no longer than 10. Try not to rest between each exercise for longer than 10 seconds. This should allow sufficient time to get into the next position. With the last isometric exercise completed, then perform a set of 10 super-slow isotonic repetitions of the corresponding isotonic shoulder exercise.

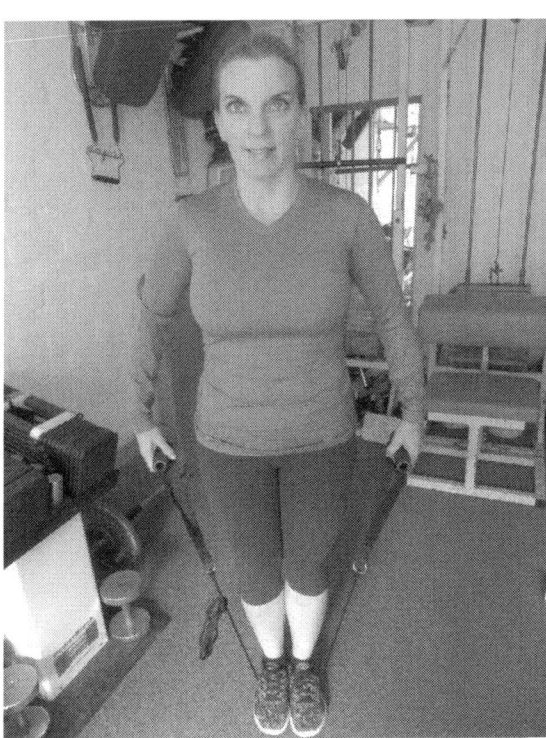

Take 10 seconds to complete the lifting phase, and 10 seconds to complete the lowering phase. Always avoid using momentum to aid the exercise.

Isometric Shoulder Exercise Example A

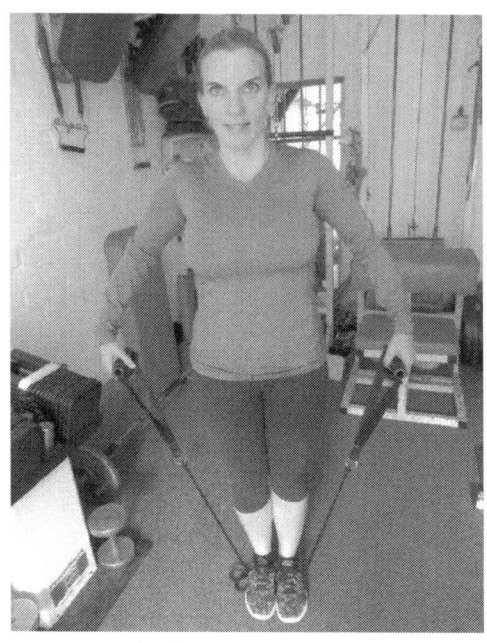

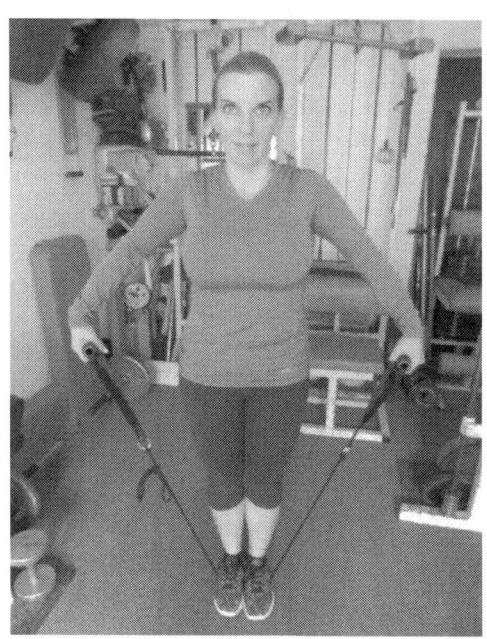

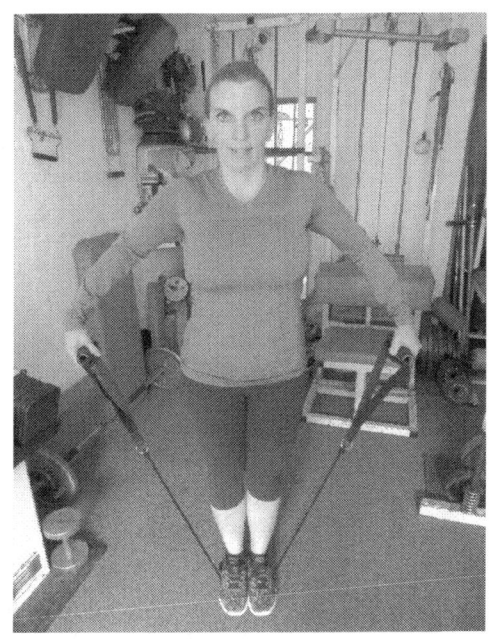

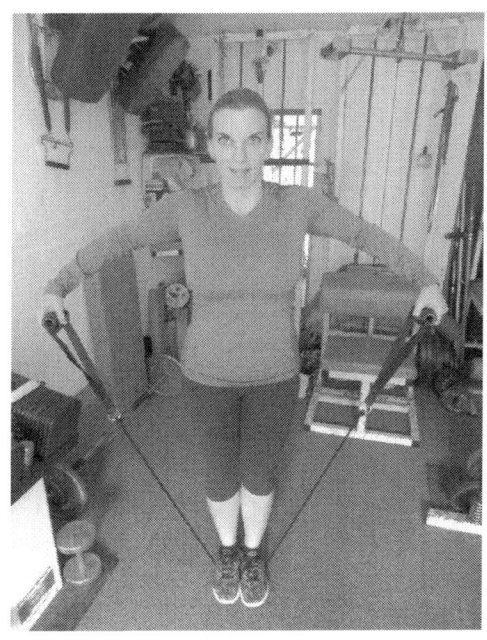

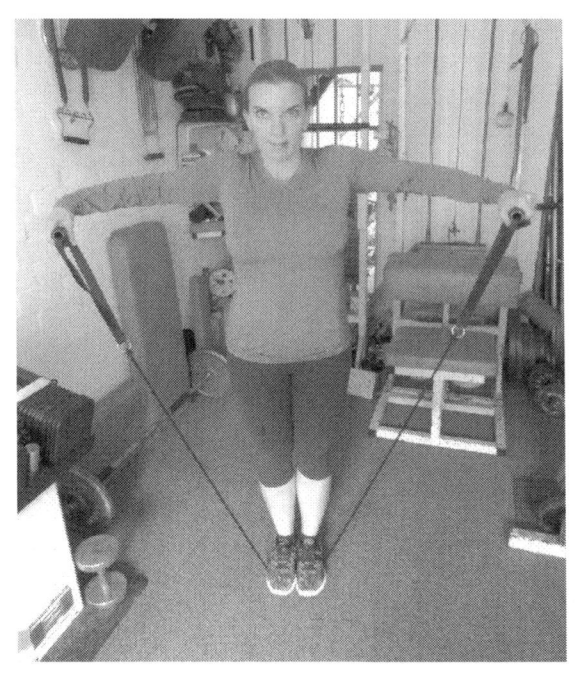

Isometric Shoulder Exercise Example B

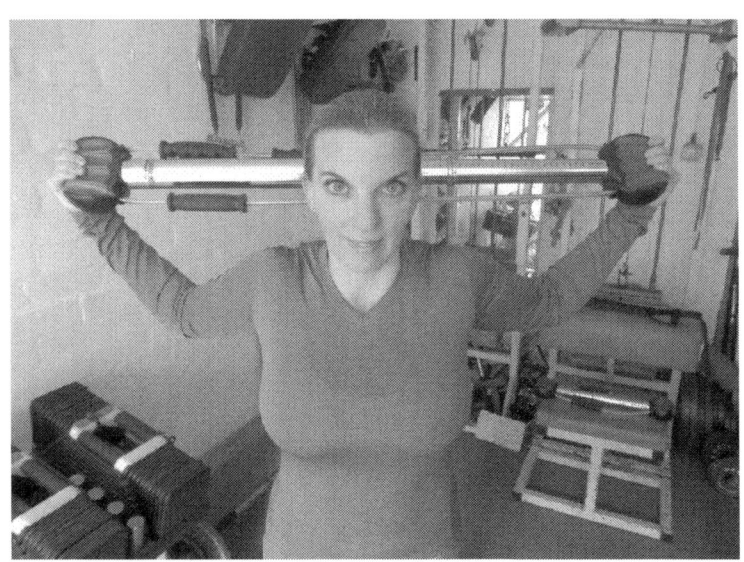

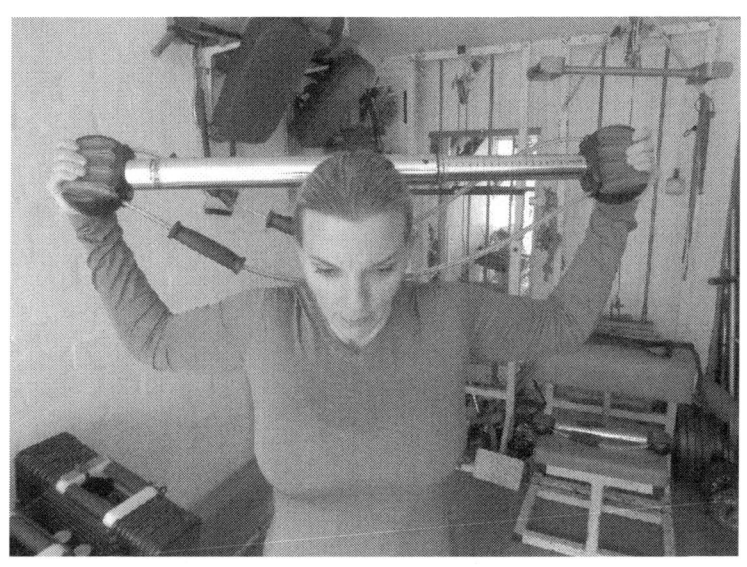

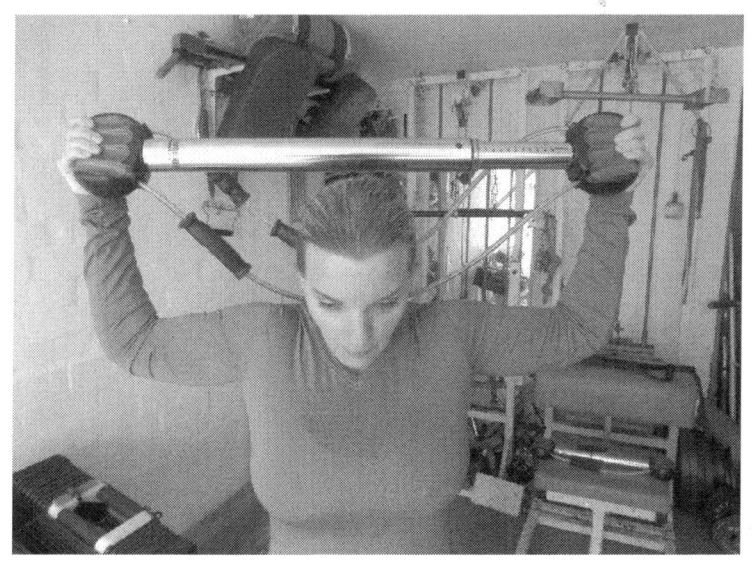

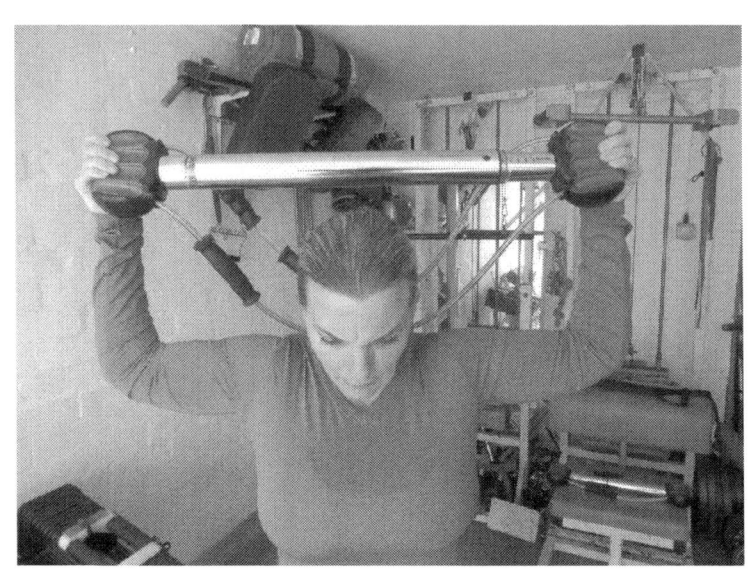

Isotonic Shoulder Exercise Example A

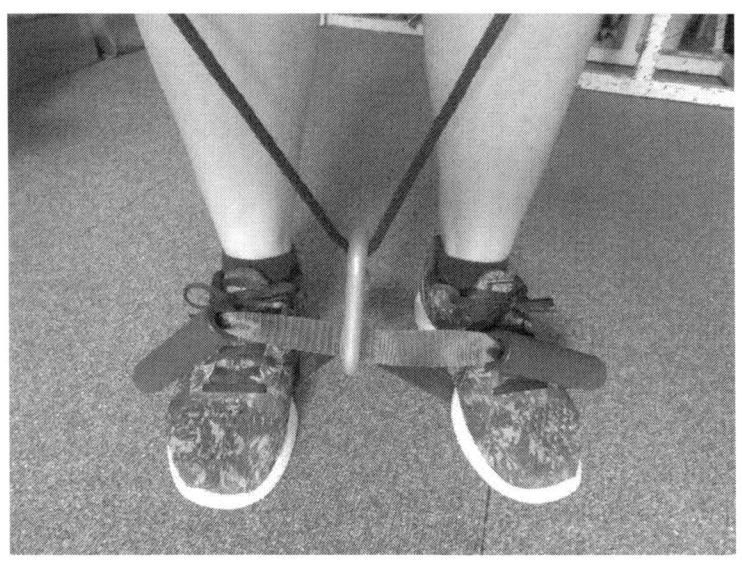

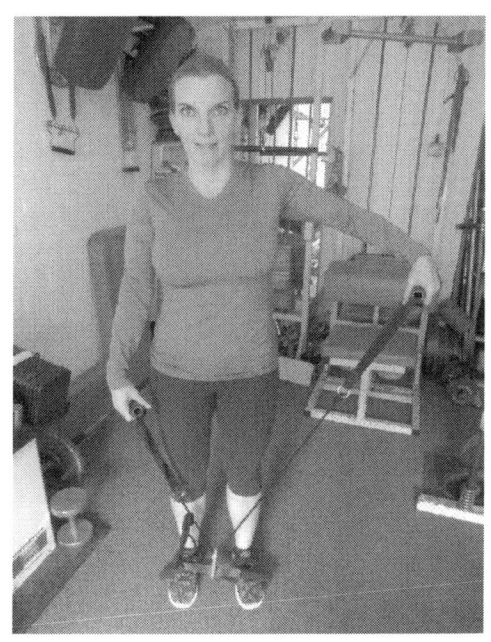

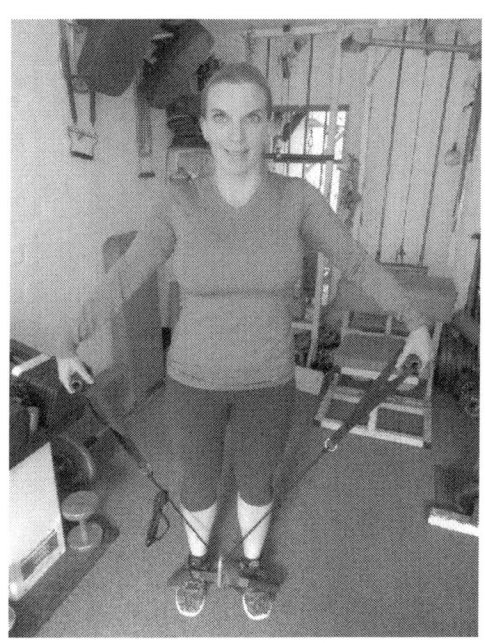

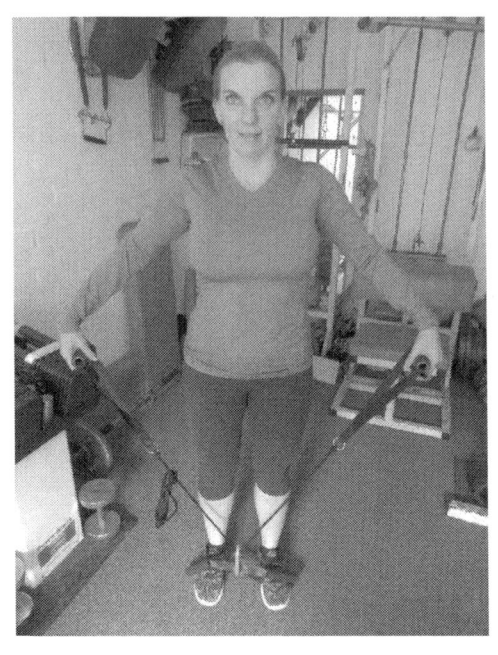

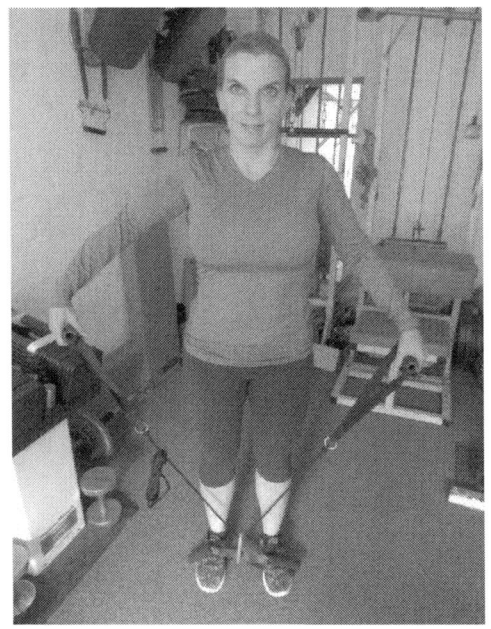

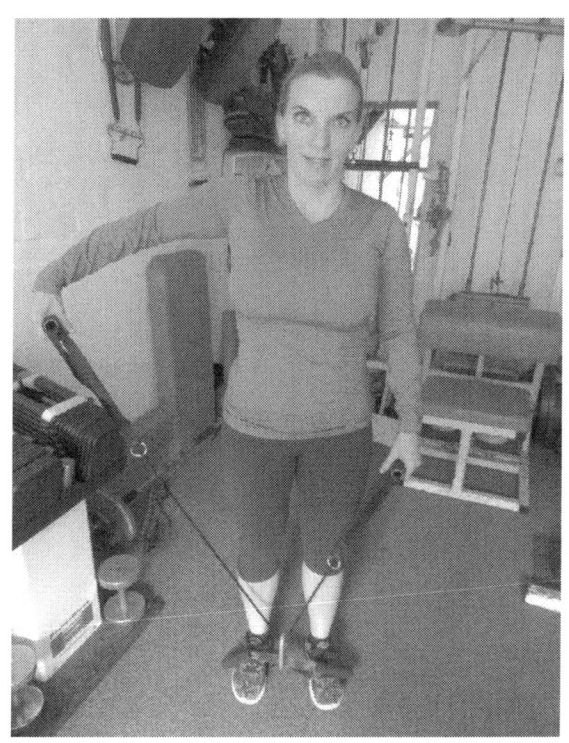

Isotonic Shoulder Exercise Example B

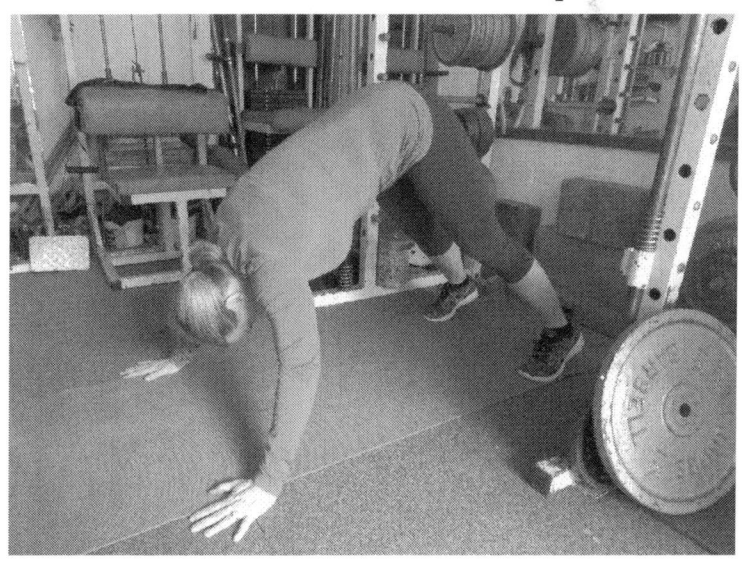

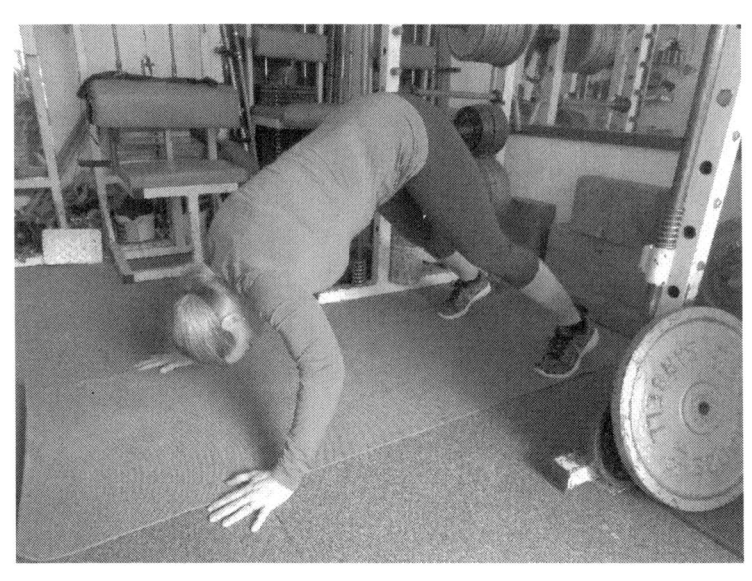

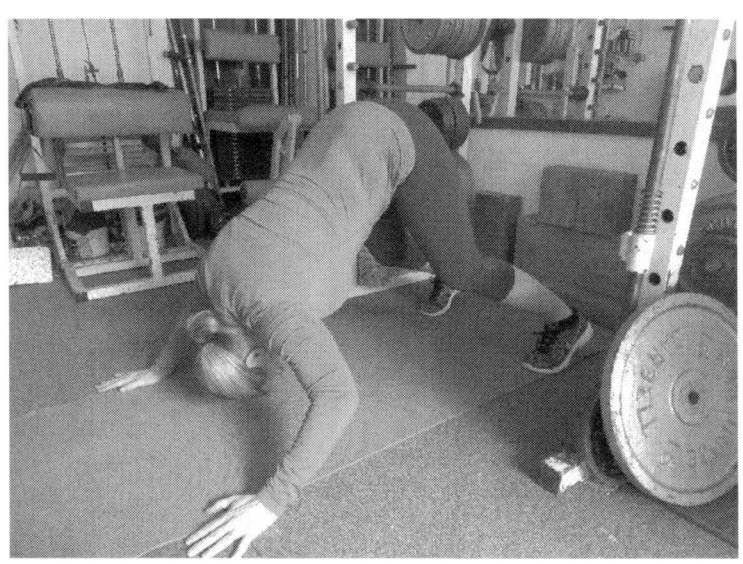

Chapter 8: Conclusion

In our world today where time is always at a premium, there's always going to be a time-crunch that's created by exercising using traditional methods. There's just no getting away from the fact that these systems take time to perform, and typically they must be performed in a gym. This then adds even more time to the crunch because you then need to add in the time needed to travel there and back to the gym, changing room hassles, and the perennial problem of having to wait for equipment to become free so that you can use it. In our modern world exercise efficiency is what it's all about. Why waste any more time exercising than you really need to? It makes no sense to do that. The TRISOmetric™ exercise system gives you total exercise efficiency. It's a science-based system that provides a high-intensity workout to gain maximum strength and muscles growth in the minimum possible time.

We already know that isometrics are extremely efficient at building great strength and muscle. We also know that isotonic exercise is extremely good at this too, albeit not quite as efficient as isometrics. The TRISOmetric™ exercise system offers the best of both worlds in a super-efficient time-saving way. Using TRISOmetric™ exercises you get maximum benefit from 3 position isometric holds to give you a smooth strength curve along the range of motion of each limb. You then also get all the additional benefits of the super-slow isotonic phase of the exercise.

As I briefly mentioned earlier, I originally developed the basis of this system back in the mid 1980's, when I was training with and coaching my old friend Jon Pall Sigmarsson. He was a great believer in isometric exercises which he believed gave him the edge he needed to win his World's Strongest Man titles. When we were training together in Finnur Karlson's gym in Reykjavik, Iceland, we were constantly on a quest to find new ways to increase our training intensity through the appliance of science. I remembered the original super-slow training concept I'd learned some years earlier and decided to try that in combination with multi-angle super-high intensity isometric exercises. Very soon we were regularly performing high-intensity isometric exercises in multiple positions before a super-slow set of an isotonic exercise. When maximum intensity and maximum resistance were combined with super-strict exercise form, the results were astounding. Jon Pall responded amazingly to this technique, and his already great strength grew even more. If you want to become as strong as possible, grow as much muscle as possible, becomes as fit as possible, all as fast as possible, then the TRISOmetric™ system is for you.

Since that time the TRISOmetric™ techniques have been refined and made more precise thanks to scientific research into both isometric and super-slow exercise methods. We now know the best positions to perform the minimum number of isometric exercises for each limb in order to get a smooth strength curve. We also now know that the science behind super-slow training is solid. If you have faith in the science of exercise, then have faith in the TRISOmetric™ exercise system. It's entirely based on solid science that really works.

www.MajorVision.com – www.TWiEA.com

Other books by Brian Sterling-Vete and Helen Renée Wuorio
The 70 Second Difference™

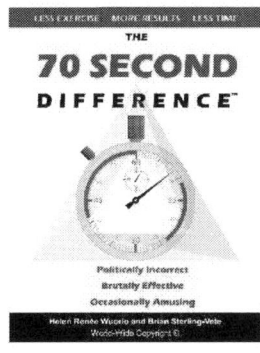

This book is a science-based no-nonsense guide that tells it straight about the most efficient ways to exercise, grow muscle, get strong and into great shape in as little as 70 seconds of scientifically proven high-intensity exercise a day. It pulls no punches about how lifestyle choices affect your body weight, health, fitness, muscle size, strength and body shape. To many, and especially those who aren't comfortable with new ideas and change, this book might be seen as being controversial. To others, it is a refreshing perspective that may not be politically correct to some people but it never fails to deliver the right message for those who want to get real results instead of wasting their valuable time. It also tells you what many commercial organisations don't what you to know, how much protein you really need, the hidden dangers of dairy products, and meats. Recommended Equipment: 2 x Iso-Bows® - available on Amazon or direct from Bullworker.com

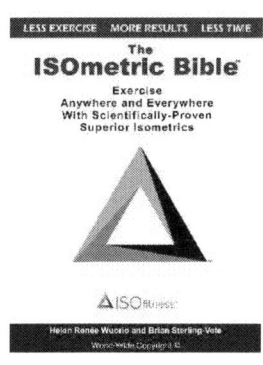

The ISOmetric Bible™ - Exercise Anywhere with Scientifically Proven Isometrics
At 335 pages, the ISOmetric Bible™ is one of the most complete, scientific, practical, and user-friendly books on isometrics that's ever been written. Isometrics have been proven by science to grow muscle and strength

faster and more efficiently than any other exercise system. It doesn't matter if you're a complete beginner, someone who's already active but wants to do more, or if you're an advanced professional athlete, everyone gets the same proportional benefits to the effort they put in. No time to exercise? Travelling away from home? Are you too busy with work commitments? With isometrics you can exercise your entire body in only minutes each day, they set you free to exercise anywhere and everywhere you choose, on a plane, in a car, or even while you're at work.   You don't need any special equipment to get a great total-body workout, but the book shows you how to use easy to find everyday objects such as walking poles, broom handles, rope and towels to exercise with. Exercise science expert Brian Sterling-Vete is a veteran exercise and strength coach and is acclaimed as one of the world's leading authorities on isometrics. Brian has trained multiple national and world champions including 2 x World Martial Arts Champion Stuart Hurst, and 4 x Times World's Strongest Man Jon Pall Sigmarsson of Iceland.

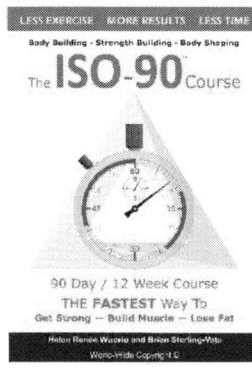

The ISO90™ Course

ISO90™ is a comprehensive and complete step by step 90-day/12-week body shaping, bodybuilding and functional strength building course based on the ISOfitness™ system of isometric exercises. The ISO90™ course is ideal for beginners, advanced trainers alike. Your natural Adaptive Response™ mechanism means that whatever intensity you apply at whatever level you're at gives everyone roughly the same percentage of improvement. The ISO90™ course focusses the appliance of science in practical exercise and functional strength building, and in doing so, it makes the ISO90™ 90-day/12-week course, one of the fastest, and most efficient ways to get into shape, build muscle, and get strong which has ever been devised. The ISO90™ course allows you to benefit from a professional-level workout literally anywhere and on almost any location. Each week will build upon the gains made in previous weeks, with clear instruction and pictures to demonstrate how each exercise should be performed. Required Equipment: 2 x Iso-Bows® - available on Amazon or from Bullworker.com

Workout at Work™

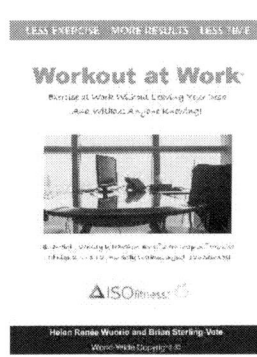

A stark new warning from the Icahn School of Medicine at Mount Sinai School of Medicine in New York reveals that sitting at a desk working for more than 6 hours a day can cause potentially irreversible damage can be done to your heart, together with increases in both cholesterol and body fat, as well as insulin resistance which is a precursor to type 2 diabetes. Even exercising 4 evenings a week after work, or for long periods over the weekend, won't fix the damage. The average person spends over 10 years of their life at work over an average 45 year working life, which can mean sitting at a desk for 10-years! There is never enough time to spare in modern life and exercising the traditional way in a gym 3-days a week, will consume a further 4.27

years. Therefore, time is the #1 reason why people don't exercise. What if you could workout effectively while you were at work? What if a complete beginner could exercise with equal ease to an advanced athlete and all without leaving your desk? Now you can do exactly that with The ISOfitness™ system of advanced isometric exercises. Even if you perform just one 7-second high-intensity exercise every 30 minutes at your desk, you'll gain maximum benefit from this scientifically proven system. At the end of a 9-hour working day you can easily perform an 18-20 exercise total-body workout leaving you healthier, fitter, stronger, and with more time to spend with family and friends. Your boss won't complain either, because in exchange for just 126 seconds out of your working day, you'll be up to 30% more efficient at your job, and you'll take less time off sick. Required Equipment: 2 x Iso-Bows® - available on Amazon or from Bullworker.com

Fitness on the Move™

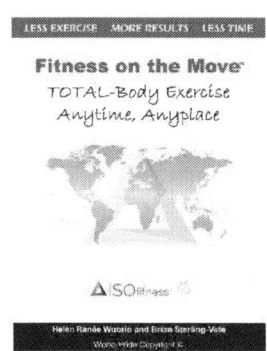

Exercising anywhere is the key to getting the most from your workouts because you'll never be confined to a gym ever again. No matter where you are, or if you're away from home for business or pleasure, you can still maintain a workout to suit all levels of fitness from beginner right up to the advanced professional athlete. The advanced isometric exercises of the ISOfitness™ system have been scientifically proven in over 5,500 independent experiments to be superior to traditional exercise methods. We've tried and tested the

Fitness on the Move™ system by performing full workout routines as passengers in cars, on trains, in cramped airline seats, on mountainsides, on beaches, and once even on the deck of a ship in a storm. The ISOfitness™ system of Fitness on the Move™ allows a full-body workout in the smallest space humanly possible thanks to our Zero Footprint Workout™ concept. Required Equipment: 2 x Iso-Bows® - available on Amazon or from Bullworker.com

The Bullworker Bible™

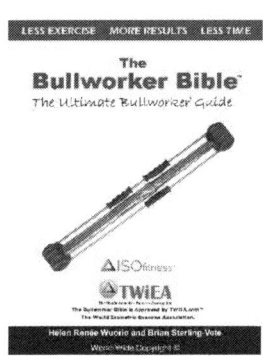

The Bullworker Bible™ is the definitive resource guide for all Bullworker® users, and it's the companion book for The Bullworker 90™ Course. The Bullworker Bible™ is approved by the makers, and distributors of The Bullworker®, at Bullworker.com and it's the complete science-based user-friendly guide of how the Bullworker® should be used properly to deliver maximum results. It also shows you how to effectively use the Bow Extension® and the Steel Bow®. It gives you all the information that you always wanted to know, but the simple wall charts and basic instruction manuals didn't provide. It tells you about Essential Repetition-Compression & Speed Control, Correct Breathing Techniques, Hooke's Law of Physics and The Bullworker®, and Correct Biomechanics for Best Results. The Bullworker Bible™ is also the essential guide for all users of the Bullworker X5, Bully Extreme, ISO 7x, and the Bullworker X7. Required Equipment: A Bullworker® Classic, or a similar device. Recommended Additional Equipment: Steel Bow®, Bow Extension® kit, 2 x Iso-Bows®.

The Bullworker 90™ Course

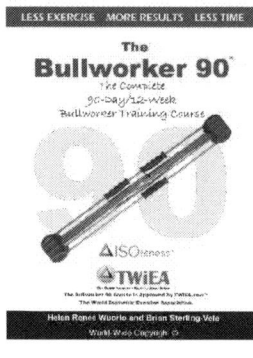

The Bullworker 90™ Course is the essential 90-day/12-week course for all Bullworker® users, and it's the companion book to The Bullworker Bible, approved by the makers, and distributors of The Bullworker®. The Bullworker 90™ is a 400+ page, science-based, user-friendly, step-by-step course designed to increase strength, fitness, grow muscle, body-build, and increase power over a 90-day/12-week period. New exercises are added almost every week, with complete routine changes every two weeks. Each week has a detailed note section, together with suggestions about exercise days, and rest times etc., so that you know exactly what to do, and when to do it. It includes Step-by-step, week-by-week instruction, progressively increasing intensity over 90 days, routine changes every two weeks, isotonic and Isometric exercise combinations, multi-angle isometric exercise combinations. The Bullworker 90™ Course can be used with the Bullworker® Classic, the Steel Bow®, the Bullworker X5, the Bully Extreme, the ISO 7x, and the Bullworker X7. The Bullworker 90™ Course also contains alternative/extra exercises which incorporate the use of the Iso-Bow®, and the Bow Extension® to increase the range and effectiveness of the device. Required Equipment: A Bullworker® Classic, or a similar device. Recommended Equipment: Steel Bow®, Bow Extension® kit, 2 x Iso-Bows®.

The Doorway to Strength - *Turn a Door into a Strength-Building Multigym.*

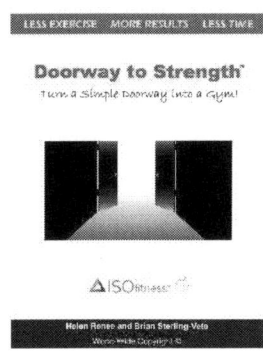

The Doorway to Strength™ shows how a simple door, doorway, and doorframe can be used to create a multi gym of exercises using the amazing Iso-Bow® exerciser and the ISOfitness™ exercise system. It demonstrates how to perform a host of powerful and effective exercises such as the door leg press and shoulder power push, together with many other exercises to work all the major body parts. The Iso-Bow® exerciser is probably the world's smallest and most powerful portable total-body exerciser. They are so small and compact even that a pair of Iso-Bows® can easily fit into the pocket of an average pair of jeans. However, just one Iso-Bow® can deliver the perfect level of workout intensity for a beginner or an advanced athlete, and with no adjustment necessary. The ISOfitness™ exercise system aims to deliver more results, in less time, and with less exercise than any other exercise system. Required Extra Equipment: 2 x Iso-Bows® (preferably 4), a solid door wedge/stop.

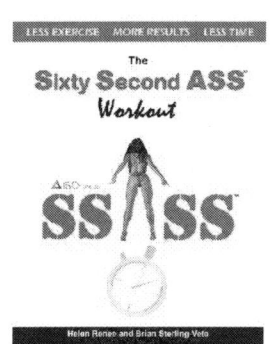

The SSASS™ Course

The Sixty Second ASS Workout™, or SSASS™ workout, is the fastest and most effective "ass" workout ever devised. Based on the scientifically proven principles of the ISOfitness™ exercise system, the SSASS™ workout is a no-nonsense, no time-wasting workout that really does do everything you need to make your ass, tight, firm, shapely, and strong. The SSASS™ routine means no more time-wasting workouts where you twist, shake, wiggle around, kick your legs, or dance around for 30 minutes, which might feel like fun but don't deliver the results you want. Everyone has 60 seconds of time to spare, even on the busiest day, so, you're Just 60 seconds a day from having a great ass. Required Equipment: 2 x Iso-Bows - available on Amazon or from Bullworker.com

Mental Martial Arts

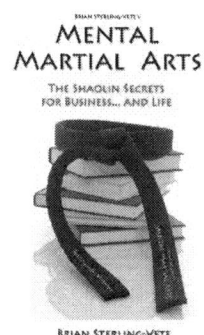

Brian Sterling-Vete's Mental Martial Arts is a system of intellectual life-combat skills which uses the tactics and principles of the physical martial arts. All interaction in life, at work and communicating with others is an exchange of energy, power and influence. One party is always exerting maximum influence over the other as they attempt to gain the outcome they prefer over the weaker party. The more powerful and persuasive will usually end as the winner, unless the apparently "weaker" person is trained in the martial arts… With this system, you can learn to verbally, intellectually, and emotionally guide, channel, and redirect the energy of others, even powerful people and large organisations. In doing so, you achieve the outcome you desire in both life and business. It also contains a specific section about how to handle a potentially hostile media in the event of a crisis. Brian combines his system of Mental

Martial Arts, together with the experience he gained in over a decade with BBC TV News, to help you and your organisation stay "Media Safe". www.mentalmartialarts.tv

Tuxedo Warriors

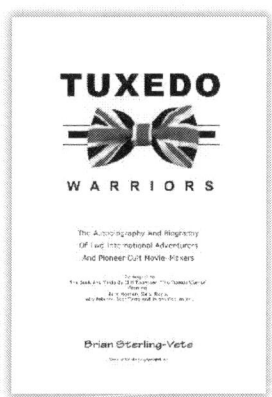

Tuxedo Warriors is the companion book to The Tuxedo Warrior book and movie, which are the autobiography of author, composer, movie-maker Cliff Twemlow. The original book ended at the beginning of what has been called the Golden Age of Video Cinematography, which he inspired. The Tuxedo Warriors is the most complete biography of Cliff Twemlow ever written. It's also the autobiography Brian Sterling-Vete, who played a central role in this unique, entertaining, and true story of two extraordinary "Renaissance-Men" and their adventures as guerrilla movie-makers. They also encountered a poltergeist when living in Iceland, and a UFO encounter which the Police also witnessed. Tuxedo Warriors continues the story where the

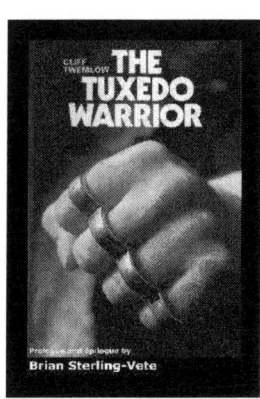

original book ends. Brian is perhaps the only person who can tell the complete story from the time it all began, right through until the end, with the sudden and untimely death of his great friend Cliff.

The Tuxedo Warrior by Cliff Twemlow – Prologue and epilogue by Brian Sterling-Vete

There are many ways in which a Doorman can gain respect. Numerous methods applied to the principal. In my profession, every available technique must be utilised, depending on the situation and circumstances. Would-be transgressors either move-off the premises quietly acknowledging your diplomatic approach. Or, the other alternative whereby physical persuasion must be exercised, which either quells their pugilistic desires, or it triggers their aggressive instincts, turning the whole incident into a bloody and violent encounter. 'The Tuxedo Warrior,' pulls no punches in its brawling, savage, colourful, and entertaining exposure of society's nightlife activities. The above is the original text from the rear cover of Cliff's book. Cliff and I were extremely close friends, and I'm honoured to re-publish his original work, which completes the storyline of my own book, 'Tuxedo Warriors.' Where Cliff's original book ends, my own book overlaps and begins, to complete his colourful life story. I'm also honoured to be close friends with his eldest son, Barry Twemlow, and sincerely thank him for enabling this book, and others that Cliff wrote, to be re-published.

The Pike by Cliff Twemlow – Prologue and epilogue by Brian Sterling-Vete

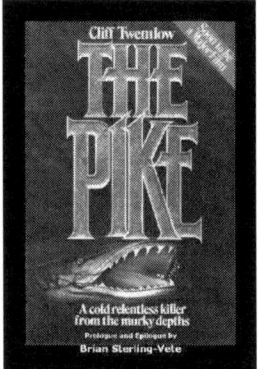

ITS FIRST VICTIMS - A screeching swan... A fisherman overboard... A drunken woman...

One by one, the mysterious killer in Lake Windermere claims its terrified victims. Tearing off limbs with its monstrous teeth, horribly mutilating bodies. Fear sweeps the peaceful holiday resort when experts identify the creature as a giant pike…. A hellish creature with the strength to rupture boats, and the anger to attack them. But for some, the terror becomes a bonanza—the traders who cater to the gathering crowds of ghouls on the shore. And, they will do anything to stop divers finding the creature. Meanwhile the ripples of bloodshed widen…. The Pike. The above is the original text from the rear cover of Cliff's book. I remember this book going into pre-production as a major movie in the early 1980's starring Joan Collins. Sadly, the financiers ran into personal difficulties and it was never made. Today, there is now renewed interest in this book as a screenplay and movie. In my own book, 'Tuxedo Warriors,' I tell the behind the scenes story of myself, my close friend Cliff Twemlow, and The Pike.

The Beast of Kane by Cliff Twemlow – Prologue and epilogue by Brian Sterling-Vete

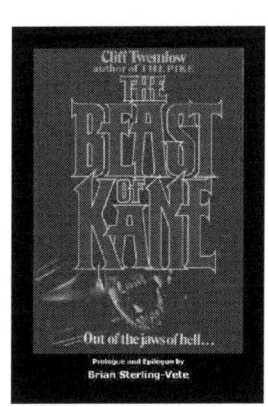

When the Gordon Family open their door to a stray Elkhound, they unwittingly welcome-in the forces of evil. For, according to the local priest, the huge dog is Satan himself, fulfilling an ancient prophecy.

But, no one will believe this warning… Even when sheep – and wolves – are mysteriously slaughtered. Even when frenzied pets turn on their owners. Even when Emily Forrest is savagely eaten alive – the first of many human victims.

As winter tightens its icy grip on the remote town of Kane, its unprotected people must face an unearthly terror.

The above is the original text from the rear cover of Cliff's book. This was the first of Cliff's books to be accepted by Hammer Film Studios to be made into a big-screen horror movie, along with Cliff's other book, The Pike. More importantly, the reason why it was never to be made into a movie was no reflection on the book itself. It was entirely because of the increasing financial challenges Hammer Films were facing at that time. They were issues that were so serious, that they caused the unexpected and rapid decline of the studio.

Paranormal Investigation - The Black Book of Scientific Ghost Hunting and How to Investigate Paranormal Phenomena

Paranormal Investigation, and especially Ghost Hunting, has long been regarded as pseudoscience and dismissed by closed-minded members of the traditional scientific community. We believe they're wrong to take this approach. Just because they currently can't detect paranormal phenomena in a laboratory, doesn't mean that it doesn't exist.

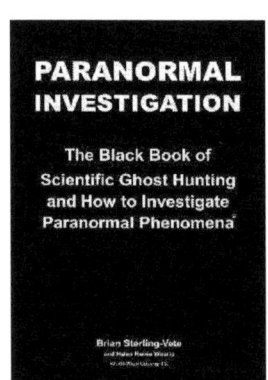

This book is an objective look at paranormal investigation. it outlines a solid scientific approach that can be used by all paranormal investigators in their research. It also contains several example stories of previously untold paranormal events which have taken place, a ground-breaking UFO sighting, and paranormally active haunted locations. It is ideal for those who are new to paranormal investigation and ghost hunting, and for more experienced investigators who want to learn more about how to apply a critical-path scientific approach. It contains a special scientific critical path graphic page to work from when devising ghost hunting experiments and to help train team members. The book also contains a step-by-step guide to a complete paranormal investigation and important information about how to protect yourself from malevolent paranormal entities that can attack you.

The Haunting of Lilford Hall - The Birthplace of the United States as a Nation Haunted by the Man Behind The Pilgrim Fathers

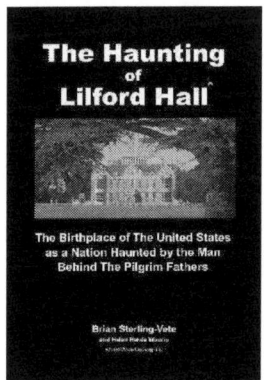

The Haunting of Lilford Hall is one of the most baffling cases of paranormal activity experienced simultaneously by multiple people ever recorded. Between 2012 and 2013, a team of 13 people came together to produce a historical TV documentary, not a paranormal investigation.

The TV documentary was about the life of Robert Browne, the man who was behind The Pilgrim Fathers sailing on The Mayflower to settle the first civilian colony on the American continent and there may never have been the United States of America, at least not as we know it today.

- Robert Browne was the man who separated church from state in the reign of Queen Elizabeth 1st which is the underpinning of the United States.
- Robert Browne's words are written into the constitution of the United States.
- Robert Browne's direct descendent officially fired the first shot in the American war of independence.
- Robert Browne's beloved Lilford Hall estate was the home of President George Washington's Mother.
- Robert Browne's beloved Lilford Hall estate was the home of President Quincy Adams' family.

Just like in a horror movie plot, the TV crew of 13 unsuspecting people were thrust into the middle of baffling and extensive paranormal activity. They experienced doors that refused to stay closed, they had debris thrown at them, they had a door silently ripped away from the hinges and doorframe while they were in the next room. There were even several recorded multi-witness apparitions of a man fitting Robert Browne's description. It is believed that the ghost of Robert Browne, the "Grandfather" of the United States as a nation, still haunts Lilford Hall to this day.

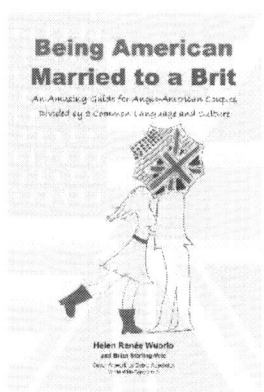

Being American Married to a Brit.

An Amusing Guide for Anglo-American Couples Divided by a Common Language and Culture

When I first started dating my British man, I never gave a second thought about differences in language and culture. Why would I?

After all, we Americans speak English, or do we...?

As dating quickly turned into being engaged, and then getting married to my British gentleman, I also found that our common language and culture was a quirky, eye-opening, and highly amusing roller-coaster ride. At times during the most basic every-day conversations, I'd be listening to his words with glazed eyes, wondering what on earth he was saying.

It really was as if we were both speaking a completely different language, even though the words that comprised the language were the same. I very quickly learned so much more about the language I was supposed to have been taught at school, the commonalities, the differences, and the good old-fashioned belly-laughs about it all that still punctuate our married life to this day.

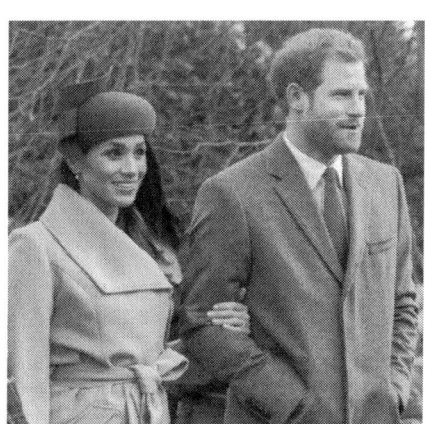

Meghan Markle and Prince Harry
Photo by Mark Jones - Wikipedia

With the Anglo-American Royal Marriage of Prince Harry and Meghan Markle, I decided to write this essential guide and dedicate it to them, and all transatlantic couples who will regularly find themselves completely divided, and confused, by their common language and culture.

www.MajorVision.com

Printed in Poland
by Amazon Fulfillment
Poland Sp. z o.o., Wrocław